A Call
to Faith

The Journey of a Cancer Survivor

J. Patrick Thomas

ISBN: 1470018462
ISBN-13: 9781470018467
Library of Congress Control Number: 2012902134
CreateSpace, North Charleston, SC

In Loving Memory of
Joe Rosenberg
Tim Betterly
David Gorham

Table of Contents

Prologue

The events that unfold before you in the life of Skip Sibley are true to the best of the author's recollections. Skip Sibley, as well as the rest of the characters in this book, have been made up in name only. The triumphs and tragedies and everyday occurrences that take place in their lives are very real.

Unfortunately, suffering is a part of life, but fortunately there is hope to counter balance the pain. Anyone who has survived cancer, lost loved ones, and witnessed family deconstruction has a story to tell. Skip Sibley is a regular guy who lived such a life. His successes are not unlike your own, and his recrudescence of difficult issues afflicts the everyday man or woman. The undercurrent of stress and mental health concerns trouble many of us, including Skip.

If we live long enough, events will transpire that we would rather not witness. All of us will go through the good and the bad that life has to offer. But they say that it is how you react to trying times that matters, not the times themselves. Perspectives change and can go in either a positive or negative direction.

The second coming of faith in the life of Skip Sibley, it is believed, allowed him the resilience necessary to fight the physical and emotional battles that came his way. Skip's salvation was transcendental and led him to a better place. Everyone must find that place, be it of secular or nonsecular means. Faith is espoused repeatedly throughout this journey because it is the author's belief that faith is the reason Skip persevered.

This is the story of Skip Sibley, but it could be your story as well.

Chapter 1

THE NEWS

May I pray for you? Five words that would forever change his life.

†

Summer in the Lowcountry was fading. The interminable heat was finally letting up on what was one of the warmest summers on record. Those blessed enough to live here know the joys of coastal living. The beach season, which usually extended from Easter until Thanksgiving, offered a plethora of outdoor activities for everyone. But tropical storms and hurricanes were always in the back of one's mind, as the warm coastal waters acted as an all-you-can-eat buffet to feed these tropical giants. Thus far, the fronts were rather noneventful, ranging from Tropical Storm Ana and Claudette that flittered with the South Carolina coastline to other storms that stayed out at sea.

The departure of the long days of summer meant shorter, but ever so glorious days of fall. As with most small southern towns, and, for that matter, most rural settings throughout the country, fall signified many things, one being the county fair. Malcolm "Skip" Sibley was constantly reminded of this October tradition. His daughter, Caroline, the older of two children in the Sibley family, made sure of it. Ashley, Skip's charming bride of over twenty years, was his high school sweetheart. They had married young, defeating the odds and defying the ever-growing divorce rate. Skip, a handsome, gregarious man who never met a soul he didn't instantly befriend, was also a small businessman in what was an entrepreneurial local economy. His MBA in finance was originally minted for Wall Street, but it would end up suiting him well in the Lowcountry business environment. Ashley was the quintessential wife who juggled marriage, family, and work. Her crystal-blue eyes and full figure were as stunning as ever, even after all those years of marriage. Skip often said, referring to the Buddhist tradition, that if he were reincarnated he would come back as a stay-at-home mom with school-aged kids, genuinely believing that his work at the office was more stressful than Ashley's work at home.

But they were far from being Buddhists. The only real religion for any true southerner in the Bible Belt was Christian. The only differentiating issue was which of the thousand sects one would adhere to. Skip and his family were faithful Christians who attended West Copper Church religiously each Sunday. While Skip carried the extra-large King James Bible with the great red-ribbon bookmark, in his heart he knew he was going through the motions, not really knowing, but like many, seeking the truth. What is the truth?

✝

"Daddy, let's ride the tea cups," bellowed Caroline Sibley, the lone daughter in the Sibley family. Caroline, five years old and a rising kindergartener, was born beautiful and grew lovelier with each passing day. Although it was said that Caroline resembled her mother, Skip believed her striking features came from the Sibley bloodline, naturally. Caroline was the kind of child that would be noticed in a crowd, as she stood in line at an ice cream shop or as she walked through the park. Skip knew his hands would be full one day with his baby girl. Not particularly good with firearms and of average weight and height, he'd have to resort to cerebral means to keep the future beaux away from his princess. Driving her to the prom and picking up her date in the company van that made a horrific beeping sound when put in reverse came to mind. Perhaps such an embarrassment would scare him off. There was also the ever-popular ritual of telling the first date that Caroline was a very slow learner who never became potty trained, hence the large-sized undergarments under her jeans. In any event, the high maintenance road would best be the one pursued by Dad.

Fall in Charleston was as picturesque as it could be. The town was actually a peninsula, bordered on the south by the Atlantic Ocean, the west by the Ashley River, and the east by the Cooper River. This was a peculiar landscape; indeed, one thinks mostly of heading east when heading to the beach if you are from the East Coast. However, Charleston was angled such that it was located on a southerly course to the shore, which actually was divided by the Intracoastal Waterway before hitting the barrier islands that fronted the sea. All in all, it was an indescribable location that morphed from a small coastal genesis to a popular seaside tourist attraction.

The beach was within a stone's throw from the Sibley residence, as the property backed up to the marshland that would eventually run into the Intracoastal Waterway, which one can travel the length of the East Coast without ever entering the ocean. With modest ocean views, a person with 20/10 vision could make out a diminutive seaside from his or her home. If they ever sold the property, Skip thought, he could work "on the water" somewhere into the real estate description. Skip decided to head up to the beach with Trovo, the family dog, to throw a ball around and take a swim in the warm October ocean. This was their evening ritual; it released Trovo's stress and gave Skip a chance to wag his tail and play fetch. As all dog owners know, their dog is the best, smartest, and the most fun playmate. "Trovo" means "found" in Latin according to Officer Rob, who helped take Trovo home the evening he was found. "Don't you love free dogs that end up costing you $12,000 in vet bills?" Skip had joked. Nothing like it.

Trovo jumped into the back of Skip's Dodge Ram pickup truck and they took the short ride over the Ben Sawyer Bridge that separates Charleston from the barrier islands and the beach. Trovo had more energy than a high school couple going at it on a Friday night.

As the throwing continued at the beach, Skip noticed that his throws to Trovo were not going as far out into the ocean as they normally did, and his arm felt a little tight. An Advil or Tylenol was in his future, he thought. Skip chalked it up to old age as he put Trovo into the back of the truck and headed home.

It seemed as if every kid in the Bay Club neighborhood, where the Sibleys had resided for some twenty years, had a basketball basket. As they passed the Gorham's house Skip saw David and his two young sons shooting hoops. The Bay Club community had its own history. The Bay Club area was a parcel of land granted to the Dodge family by the King of England in the early eighteenth century. Asparagus was the main crop grown in the area, with wild sprouts still noticeable to this day. The coastal region was also a thriving seaport at the time. The agrarian society that was Charleston utilized a series of berms, which were dirt mounds built into the creeks that led to deep water where produce was loaded onto a boat destined to ports around the world.

When Skip pulled over and Trovo jumped out, the two-versus-two game was on. David and his son Joshua took on Skip and Jacob, the other boy. It was a fun game for all, but the David and Joshua team was triumphant. During the course of the game, Skip made his way to the free-throw line several times but, each time he attempted a foul shot, it came up woefully short. Again Skip wrote it off to sore muscles and the fact that he was approaching forty years of age; but that had never happened before.

✝

As a kid, Skip associated the fair with cotton candy and rides like most other kids, but for him it was also a place where an underage kid could gamble legally. Sure, he remembered the tubs-of-fun and the Himalaya rides. He also recalled the usually stoned teenager who operated the shoddily put together ride playing a song from the Edgar Winter Band, and barking, "Do you want to go a little faster?" But mostly he remembered the games. Not the ones for stuffed animals or Atlanta Braves hats, but the ones that actually returned drachma. Skip was drawn to the roulette wheels and dice games among several others, where a modicum of skill—but mostly luck—decided your financial fortune.

The normal summer employment for young Skip was mowing lawns in the neighborhood for about ten dollars an hour—not fun in August when the heat index hovered around 190 degrees! The idea of making money, however, was lodged in the back of Skip's head at an early age, which, he eventually realized, is probably how he wound up in the financial markets on Wall Street.

†

Caroline was insistent that they hit the rides first at the Lowcountry Carolina Fair. However, memories of his youth danced in his head and beckoned Skip toward the gaming area, but what kind of example would that set for his young daughter with those bright green innocent eyes? Skip acquiesced, and they headed in the general direction of the moving attractions where they stumbled upon what looked like a ride he called the "spider" when he was young, a contraption that looked like it was assembled by a dozen monkeys in under fifteen minutes. The only thing that held riders in their seat—and from certain death—was a small cotter pin that looked like something that fell off a Barbie doll. "Caroline, are you sure you want to ride this thing? It looks a little scary, even to me." Being all of five and fearless, she insisted they get in line and ride the beast. After what seemed like an eternity in line on the fair's first Saturday night, it was finally their turn to venture aboard. Caroline raced in first and got the inside seat of the two-seater, which was fine with Skip because looking at the design of the ride, it seemed safer for her to sit on the inside. Caroline sat down and Skip followed. The ride was about to start. Skip put his right arm around the back of Caroline to comfort her and hold her in place but, as he lowered his right arm around Caroline's shoulder, they heard a horrible sound. An odd, unrecognizable sound. A sound that not only manifested unimaginable pain, but a sound that brought forth the promise that his life was never again to remain the same. What kind of father would leave a five-year-old alone on a ride as it was about to start?

✝

It was time. The Cesarean section for baby number two was about due. With unwavering fears of childbirth, this Southern Belle knew of only one true way to bring a precious new life into the world: with an epidural and a planned "C" section. Skip was more old-fashioned, growing up in a large family and being the eldest, remembering the stories his father told of his mother screaming in agony while giving birth to his younger siblings. Ah, the inequities that woman must still contend with from Eve's original sin. I don't think Ashley will eat an apple to this day.

All was proceeding as normal. Mom was sufficiently numb, and Skip was in the waiting room with the other Dads, also sufficiently numb, watching the Braves get clobbered by the Mets. After one World Series title, the men thought that they should be able to reproduce it every year. As Greg Maddux was going into his windup, the nurse came out and told Skip that it was time. Up and at 'em. As Skip and the nurse approached Ashley's room, the most horrific sounds of terror were bellowing from the room next door. In wonderment, and against the nurses' wishes, Skip stuck his head in the room to see what was going on. A large black woman was the one screaming, and one could not blame her, as it seemed that child after child was being pulled out of the bewildered and anguished mother. Skip would later learn that the woman had had triplets, and no epidural, explaining much of the situation. Moving on, there were more important events at hand. It was time for young Mr. Sibley to witness the birth of the baby yet to be named, number two. But good things come to those who wait. Ashley needed to know the sex of the child months ahead of time so her mother could get busy making sheets, drapes, blankets, and whatever else the two deemed essential. Again, in the tradition of men in his family before him, it was time to cut the cord—and learn whether it was a boy or girl. In typical family tradition, Skip about fainted when Dr. Lowry gave him the umbilicutter. In the most gracious way, Skip told Dr.

6

Lowry that although he went to school for six years, he was not a medical doctor and waived his obligatory right to cut the cord. No matter. Baby boy "no-name" was born healthy with five fingers and five toes on each foot and hand. Mother, father, and baby were all fine and were eventually transferred from the operating room into a room on the third floor. Skip wondered why they were in a private room (they cost more, you know), but Ashley had ordered it so that they could be alone and not disturbed upon arrival.

Skip remembered, as most Dads do, that no matter whether it is your first child or your fifth, it is one of the proudest and most profound moments in life. Looking through the glass, he wondered what would become of his new introduction to the world. Time travels fast during these first few hours and days at the hospital. Whether one believes in God or not, one prays that, more than anything, this child will be healthy.

Skip spent the night at the Trident Hospital with Ashley to keep her company and to take a break from the rest of the family at the house, which was fortuitous. At four o'clock in the morning, a doctor walked into their room with a look on his face that said anything other than, "Have you given the new baby a name yet?" The doctor was not Dr. Lowry, who delivered their child, but a pediatric cardiologist. Ashley and Skip grew tense together as the doctor told them that on a routine examination of the baby, it was discovered he had a hole in his heart. Congenital heart defects, the doctor said, are abnormalities in the heart's structure that can be present at birth. Approximately eight out of every one thousand newborns have congenital heart defects, ranging from mild to severe. The baby had a Ventricular Septal Defect (VSD), a defect in the septum between the right and left ventricles. In most people, the cause isn't known, but genetic factors may play a role. Just what the young couple with a new baby wants to hear— that their child has a potentially serious heart condition. The news was devastating and threw Ashley and Skip into a whirlwind of concern. It was as if Skip had been plagued with a dissociative disorder where he heard the news circulating around him but felt as if he were tethered above, trying to understand why everyone was so upset. In hindsight, this is what probably set in motion a series of serious mental issues that would torture Skip for years to come.

†

As Caroline sat buckled in, waiting for the ride ready to commence, her father left the ride in a state that a five-year-old could only understand as urgent. Skip was in pain. It was off the Richter scale. He was descending into one of the lower nine layers of Dante's Inferno. When the suffering would end, only God knew. His right arm appeared broken. In the minor maneuver of placing his arm around Caroline, the weight of his arm alone was enough to cause a snap in the bone and sent Skip running, which was the only thing he could think to do. Other parents on the ride must have wondered why this guy would leave his child alone on a wild ride by herself. Coincidentally, in his stumbling efforts, he ran into Ashley's dad, who had seen the whole event unfold. A man of action, Andy Foster grabbed Caroline from the ride, picked Skip up, and started the process of getting the group to the local emergency room.

It was a Sunday in the small town of Abbeboro. Few people were at the hospital, so Andy had his pick of front-row parking spots. By this time, word had spread to family and friends that the group was on its way to the emergency room to have Skip checked out. Andy was pretty sure Skip broke his arm and would need it set, so this was the message the Sibley family received. Skip was the only patient of the young doctor on duty in the emergency room that Sunday afternoon. His name was Joseph Lardy. Dr. Lardy, who couldn't have been more than thirty years old, was doing a sports medicine rotation through the hospital. He could see that Skip was in pain, so he ordered the compulsory round of blood work and x-rays. The young doctor put Skip through a regimen of painful arm movements in an attempt to discern the problem.

Skip's blood work came back fine and, with no radiologist on duty, young Dr. Lardy read the x-ray himself. Skip had guessed that since this hospital was a long way from the Mayo Clinic, Dr. Lardy probably hadn't had much exposure to reading x-rays or performing emergency room work.

As it turned out, he was here for several weeks while on this sports medicine rotation and would soon be whisked off somewhere else. At first, Dr. Lardy could find nothing wrong with Skip's arm or shoulder and was baffled as to why Skip appeared to be in such serious pain. "I just don't see anything; I'm not sure what's going on here" was what he kept repeating.

Ashley's mother, a nurse who worked for a physician's office located next door to the hospital, often made rounds at the hospital and knew most of the folks who worked there. As fate would have it, one of the doctors from the practice, Dr. Stuben, a brilliant Harvard-educated physician in his late fifties, happened to be visiting one of his patients in the hospital on his normal Sunday afternoon rounds. He noticed Andy in the emergency room waiting area. After they exchanged pleasantries, Dr. Stuben asked why Andy was at the emergency room and not on the golf course, which is where one would normally find the scratch golfer on a beautiful Sunday afternoon. Andy briefly recounted the tale to Dr. Stuben of young Dr. Lardy's perplexity in this diagnosis. Without hesitation, Dr. Stuben headed toward the emergency room to look at the x-ray himself. It took only a moment before he noticed the small, scallop-shaped indentions on the humerus bone.

Not only was Dr. Stuben an excellent surgeon, but he was also a man of God and had a heart that had been given to God. Born Jewish, Dr. Stuben was now a Messianic Jew, combining elements of Judaism and Christianity into a single faith. By this time Skip, Ashley, Andy, and Caroline were all present in the emergency along with Dr. Stuben. Dr. Stuben looked at Skip and, without missing a beat, asked him if he had ever had cancer before. *Cancer.* The now-familiar dissociative disorder had once again removed Skip from reality. Bewildered, Skip weighed what the doctor had just said. Pain does not fall into any one of Dante's layers, although suffering is intertwined throughout. Allegorically, Skip was discovering that it was not just mortal pain that was imprisoning him; it was that true hell is an eternal separation from God. Was Skip headed in this direction? Holding hands, everyone formed a circle. "May I pray for you?" asked Dr. Stuben.

✝

After prayers from family and friends, the baby now named Foster had recovered completely from the VSD. He also overcame a slight case of jaundice that required his remaining in the hospital for a few days longer than expected.

Chapter 2

LIFE CUT SHORT

†

On May 27, 1958, one of the finest air weapons ever used by the Navy and Marine Corps—the McDonnell Douglas F-4 Phantom II—had its first flight. It became operational in the latter part of 1960 and, by the end of 1965, many Navy and Marine squadrons were flying the Phantom II. While the primary role of the F-4 was as an interceptor, its secondary job was to provide tactical air support, so it carried a wide range of external ordnance. In addition to air attacks, the Marine Corps established the **H** (helicopter) **R** (transport) S (Sikorsky), or HRS series, as the first significant step in building a Marine Corps helicopter transport capability.

It was a cool October morning when First Lieutenant Patrick Sibley and Second Lieutenant Bobby Icle took the helm of their UH-34D helicopter for a routine training mission that would take them from Langley Air Force Base down to Charleston, South Carolina, and then back to Langley. The mission was anything but routine.

✝

After being released from Abbeboro Hospital with arm in sling and prescriptions to fill, Skip and the family drove back to Andy's house to hunker down and come up with a game plan. Ashley returned from the CVS drugstore shortly after with a container of painkillers the size of a vitamin bottle. Judging by the amount of drugs being brought his way, Skip realized that this might be more than he bargained for. The pain was terrible, but it was getting worse. He couldn't get comfortable. Lying down was out of the question, so the armchair was his initial option for rest. As Skip drifted in and out of hard-core painkiller consciousness, whispers circulated in the house about the nature of the illness and the gravity of the problem.

✝

Patrick Sibley graduated near the top of his class at Bethesda Chevy Chase High School in the Maryland suburbs of Washington, DC. He went through Quantico and became an officer in the Marines. At the young age of twenty-one, and armored with good looks, manners, and charm, Patrick prepared for a life as a Marine aviator. Patrick married his high school sweetheart, Maria Celia, and within three years had two children: the oldest a son and the youngest a beautiful daughter. Patrick began flight school in Pensacola, Florida, on the HUS helicopter. The HUS, later known as the UH-34D, became the principal vehicle in the rotary-wing lift capability of the Corps. Known to all but those who flew it, the HUS was a dangerous aircraft. In military jargon, such issues are referred to as "shortfalls in its performance parameters." Despite its shortcomings, it would be the helicopter of choice from this point in time through the Vietnam War.

✝

At this point, if anyone would have told Skip what the next several years would bring, he would have probably thrown in the towel. Skip was a good and honest person, but like Moses or Job of the Bible, Skip was not particularly confident, nor did he feel equipped with the internal strength he would need in the fight yet to come. Would it not be easier to let go and touch the Savior's hand, allowing the pain to come to an end?

When Skip began to come out of the drug-induced condition that his body had been in for some four or five hours, the gravity of the situation began sinking in. He thought he remembered hearing the word "cancer" at some point and wondered why there was an abundance of concern regarding his condition. Skip recalled with clarity, in the back of his mind, his mother-in-law, Rodine Foster, saying, "They do wonders with prostheses these days." Again, it was sensory overload, and the synapses were not nearly firing on all cylinders. Pain was all that he knew. The drugs were of some help, but nothing could really take the edge off the constant pain. A local family friend and pharmacist visited the Foster house, and the conversation that he had with Skip was striking; it was one that would resonate with Skip. It was the way that Dr. Loyd kept speaking in the past tense, as if Skip was gone or would be gone shortly. Rest. Must rest. Tomorrow will be another day.

✝

What must it be like to raise two children alone?

✝

The pre-flight checklist as required in the Corps Aviation wing was being stepped through with due diligence. All pilots must perform these checks before any flight, whether it was a training mission or going into battle. While Lieutenant Sibley was going through the pre-flight navigational routine in the cockpit, Second Officer Icle was performing the visual maintenance of the aircraft. Icle began in the cockpit with tests of the radio and the throttle as well as all pushrods and servos to make sure the swash plate was moving as it should. Icle then moved outside the aircraft for a visual inspection of basic hardware: nuts and bolts, wiring, belt tension, and mounting. Sibley motioned to Icle that the flight plan had been approved and they were ready for takeoff. All checks had been performed, so both officers entered the aircraft for takeoff. The flight from Langley to Charleston would take approximately two and a half hours at the rate of speed the crew would be flying that day. Although Charleston was a coastal city, the route would take the pilots over the piedmont sections of mostly rural North and South Carolina before heading east toward the coast. Something was bothering Icle as the flight took the helicopter over rural North Carolina around the Greensboro area. A sinking feeling began in Icle's stomach when he realized he had neglected the last of the safety checks, as he was distracted by Sibley's giving him the all-is-ready sign. The inspection of the blades and flybar was routine, but nonetheless, Icle, a man of micro orientation, couldn't help but feel that overlooking anything on the pre-flight checklist, let alone the blades, was not acceptable. He made no mention of this to First Lieutenant Sibley.

✝

Ewing's sarcoma is a degenerative cancer that usually strikes children and young adults. The peak ages for those with this rare cancer are between ten and twenty years, but younger children and older adults can also acquire Ewing's sarcoma. Sometimes referred to as PNET, Ewing's sarcoma is a cancer that can start in the bone or in soft tissues. The most common sites for Ewing's sarcoma are the pelvis, the thigh, and the trunk of the body. It is not known exactly what kind of cell gives rise to Ewing's sarcoma. Some of its features resemble the early cells that would normally develop into part of the nervous system. Nor is it known what causes Ewing's sarcoma; the most common early signs of this disease are pain and swelling. Like other sarcomas, Ewing's sarcoma can spread to other parts of the body. Even when the tumor is detected at a very small size, there may be evidence of microscopic spread. For this reason, Ewing's sarcoma always requires treatment to the whole body, which includes chemotherapy. Chemotherapy is intended to destroy any tumor cells that have spread to the rest of the body and to shrink the main mass of tumor cells. Successful treatment also requires another form of treatment to the main mass of the tumor. This can be surgery, radiation therapy, or a combination of the two. Several months would pass before Skip realized this was his fate.

†

The trip from Abbeboro back to Charleston was tense and painful. Ashley drove while she tended to the needs of a one-month-old baby, a five-year-old child, and a badly hurt husband. What would normally be a three-to-four-hour drive turned twice as long with myriad stops needed for both father and children. Skip's arm rested in a temporary cast/sling, and he was fully dosed with pain medication, but his comfort level was still extremely low. Foster was a good baby as far as one-month-old car riders go. During the drive, there was little talk about the current situation or future issues. Ashley was generally a positive individual with an ever-optimistic outlook. However, she was bombarded with worry and concern for Foster. And what about Skip? Ashley knew, after discussing the situation with the doctors and her mother and family, that Skip had at best a 50/50 chance of living. What about insurance and her job? How would she handle everything alone? Neither Skip nor Ashley had family in the area and were left to basically fend for themselves in Charleston.

Back at home in Charleston, Ashley quickly went to work setting up a network of support. She began with the neighbors. Bay Club, their small neighborhood, was a close-knit community of some two dozen residents. All but a few of the families were born and raised in Charleston, with some actually acquiring their property through a land grant via King George of England dating back hundreds of years. As one might expect, it was an arduous Sibley household. The next-door neighbor, Margaret Brown, organized daily meal preparation for the family, with each of the neighbors taking a day and a meal. This would make daily life significantly more manageable for Ashley, alleviating the challenge of fixing three meals a day. Albeit a major help, this was just the tip of the iceberg of aid the family needed. Where to begin? It was all happening so fast. The family was so young. Would God give them just as much as they could handle? Why were some given seemingly more? Was it better to suffer as the Apostle Paul had said, who noted that only in suffering are we truly close and dependent upon God? Did the Sibleys have more than they could handle? Only time would tell.

†

In an instant it was over. The main rotor blade separated from its shaft and cut horizontally across the cockpit of the helicopter. The metal of the roof was severed as a knife going through butter. Icle and Sibley disconnected from the rest of the craft and spiraled out of control toward the North Carolina soil. What took place those last few minutes before they hit the ground is not known. There were no black boxes in those days with voice recordings from the cockpit. The autopsy results indicate that they were alive until they hit the ground. What must it have been like? What had Second Lieutenant Icle been thinking? Would it have made a difference? The coroner's report listed the cause of death for both Marine pilots as a broken neck.

And then there were three: Maria, Skip, and Jacqueline. First Lieutenant Patrick Sibley was given a twenty-one gun salute with family, friends, and members of the Corps present at the funeral. A new chapter in their lives had begun.

†

It was anything but routine, but a daily routine was beginning. Ashley was the workhorse of the family. So much had to be done. It was difficult to rank the priorities that required her daily assessment.

Employment. Without work, there would be no income. Ashley worked for one of the only "white-collar" employers in the Charleston region. Everything employment-wise in the region was, for the most part, service sector-oriented or small entrepreneurial ventures. Along with the big business came the big benefits: pay, healthcare, vacation, maternity leave, and so on. But with big business also comes the downside. The corporation demands time; one's first priority must be to them. This was true at the utility company where Ashley worked. An MBA graduate from Georgetown in finance and investments, Ashley was overqualified for many jobs in the company, but she was transferred to a technology division that was somewhat foreign to her. As such, work must be done to get up to speed to make the grade expected by management, all in the name of the Holy Grail, which would be the company's latest quarterly financial report. Although Ashley had little to do with the revenues and expenses, she was aware of the ever-present pressure to perform at the highest level. Whether this job was heaven or hell had yet to be determined.

†

The p53 gene, like the Rb gene, is a tumor suppressor gene; its activity stops the formation of tumors. If a person inherits only one functional copy of the p53 gene from the parents, he or she is predisposed to cancer and usually develops several independent tumors in a variety of tissues in early adulthood. A rare condition, it is known as Li-Fraumeni syndrome. However, mutations in p53 are found in most tumor types, and so contribute to the complex network of molecular events leading to tumor formation.

The rationale behind this biological mystery was being explained to Skip and Ashley by a doctor of genetic oncology. You see, this was not the first tumor that Skip had had in his life. When he was twenty-nine years old, during a routine physical examination, a small lump was found in his throat about the size of a peppercorn. The attending internist immediately sent Skip to an ear, nose, and throat oncologist to evaluate the lump. Skip had mentioned to the doctor that he and Ashley had recently been married and were taking a honeymoon abroad for several weeks. So, the biopsy needed would be postponed until their return from Europe. The doctor already had a good idea about the results, but the humanist in him told him that the discussion could wait.

†

Life for Maria Sibley and her two young children would be difficult now that her Marine husband had died tragically. Although she had previously been employed in several top secretarial positions with the local ABC and NBC television affiliate stations in Washington DC, the births of Skip and

Jacqueline led quickly to her becoming a full-time, stay-at-home mom. The sudden loss of her young husband overwhelmed her so, when the opportunity to move back home with her parents presented itself, Maria gladly accepted.

Dominic and Mimi Celia welcomed Maria and her two small children with open arms and hearts. Dominic was a first-generation immigrant from Italy who came to America with two cousins and a friend in 1916. What had it been like to leave his home and his country at the tender age of fourteen, to journey to a new land with nothing but the clothes on his back? To Skip, "Poppop," as Dominic was known to the children, was a real hero and role model. Like most immigrants to America at the time, Dominic was young and had no real skill set to apply to the working world. As such, he was lucky enough to become a tailor apprentice at a clothing shop in Washington, DC, known as Visic Brothers. Young Dominic would eventually take to the trade and become one of the best and most popular tailors in the nation's capitol. Dominic would make suits and other clothes for everyone from athletes to famous politicians and local businessmen. Dominic, slightly heavy for his somewhat diminutive stature, was living the American dream, purchasing a home in the nearby suburbs of Bethesda, Maryland. The small brick home was in a lovely neighborhood within walking distance to schools and shops.

Words cannot describe Mimi. She was part saint and part matriarch in a domestic sense. The relationship between Mimi and Poppop was very old country. Dominic took care of work and the family finances, and Mimi took care of the home, never learning to drive. Mimi was a petite woman with long, flowing blond hair that she usually wore up in a bun. She was the kindest person that one would ever meet, and would do anything for anyone.

The Celia residence was about to double in size from three to six, as Maria and the kids were moving in. Dominic and Mimi also had a son, Maria's brother Dominic, Jr., known as Donnie. He was eleven years younger than his sister Maria and was in his teens at the time of the turbulence. He was and still is one of the funniest people one will ever meet. The house originally was barely large enough to accommodate Mimi, Poppop, and Donnie and, now Maria, Skip, and Jacqueline were added to the mix. So an addition was built at the back of the house on both the first and second levels. The top was used as another bedroom, which was occupied by Donnie, and the first floor was a den and sitting area to give added space and to make sure Poppop had plenty of room to stretch out and smoke his Pall Mall cigarettes. In that neighborhood in those days, most of the houses had basements, this one included. It was used as a second kitchen and additional recreational and storage area. And life went on.

Chapter 3

GLORY DAYS

†

The trip to Europe was a late honeymoon for Skip and Ashley that was pursuant to Skip's selling his first business that was involved in the financial markets. During the mid-1980s, with the Gordon Gekko mantra of "Greed is Good," Skip and several associates from graduate school at the American University began a small mergers and acquisitions boutique. All involved initially were in their twenties with freshly minted law and MBA degrees and were ready to conquer the world.

The trip to Europe was Skip's second. The first go around, in which Skip and several friends backpacked and Euro-railed their way around much of the continent, followed his graduation from business school. And, as would be expected from a group of twenty-somethings, they were at times boisterous and hedonistic. With nicknames like Jump, Bone, and Ski, it is no wonder they took Europe by storm and probably further contributed to the notion of the "ugly American."

The trip with Ashley, however, was much shorter and done a tad bit more on the haute couture. Although backpacking was still involved, a slightly higher quality of residence and gourmet was employed. Throughout their adventure and honeymoon, Skip hadn't the slightest notion that a storm in the form of a malignancy was forming on the horizon.

✝

Three young entrepreneurs barely out of graduate school with not much more than the shirts on their backs ventured into uncharted waters in the fast and furious game of mergers and acquisitions. It was a rollercoaster ride that would bring a modicum of fame and fortune to the still-young pups. The business concept was originally missioned to create a risk arbitrage boutique that would invest in companies that were being taken over or purchased by other companies. It was part finance and part smoke and mirrors. But the trio had a small problem: a lack of money. Mark Rosenberg was fresh out of the gates of the Washington School of Law at the American University where he and Skip met while Skip was pursuing his MBA in finance at the Kogod College of Business Administration. The third spoke in the original wheel was Phillip Lexington, an intellectual and the brains of the outfit. Mark had the idea of creating the trading shop, and he and Phillip had come together while working for the same firm located at the Securities and Exchange Commission (SEC). You see, the SEC was the repository for all information on corporate takeovers, and in those days it was the first place that private information went public. Slightly battle-scarred in their lack of ability to raise money to become a risk arbitrage trading firm, they thought that they could instead interpret the takeover information at the SEC and sell that information to other mergers and acquisition firms and risk arbitrage shops in New York and elsewhere. It was the beginning of something beautiful, at least financially speaking.

Skip and Phillip, a throwback to the '60s with long hair, a beard, and liberal leanings, worked out of the SEC and began their assault on the mountains of information in order to find those few grains of salt that could make them and others money. Mark was smart and had the gift of debate and sales, and he hit Wall Street running. He was also an accomplished wrestler and even won a gold medal at the Israeli Olympics. After several months of creating a system at the SEC to analyze the data, Mark had made five trial sales in New York, which were mergers and acquisition departments of large investment banks and brokerage firms. Mark had agreed to give the five accounts a free, three-month trial of access to the work they were doing, after which they would discuss how to proceed. It just so happened that this period in the mid-1980s was one of the hottest moments in the history of mergers and acquisitions in the United States. During the next several months in M&A, many deals were being put on the table. The dissemination of information on the deals—better known as 13Ds (named after its code under the Williams Act)—was rather archaic, even for that time. You have to understand that anytime an investor buys at least a 5 percent stake in a publicly traded company, like Walmart or IBM, the investor must file what is known as a 13D stating the number of shares purchased and the purchase price. In addition, investors must disclose their intentions regarding their shares, and possibly with the company. As basic supply and demand dictates, purchasing shares in a company generally drives up the demand for those limited shares, thereby driving up the price and, hence, the interest to the investor.

Every hour on the hour, an SEC employee pushed to the SEC conference room a grocery cart filled with 13Ds and other Williams Act filings. The documents were dropped off at a clerk's desk, and then the games began. At least half a dozen law firms and others, like Skip's company, were vying for access to the documents and the potential nuggets of gold within them. Always trying to get a leg up on the competition, Skip would befriend the SEC clerk who pushed the cart down from the fifth floor via an elevator to the first floor to the public reference room. Louis something-or-other was his name, and he was touched with some type of mental illness. Skip would occasionally ride the elevator down with Louis, making small talk and peaking out of the corner of his eye at the bounty of documents. Louis would always scold Skip if he caught him eyeing those documents. It was all just a lot of fun until the documents were delivered to the clerk's desk in the public reference room. At that time, if a layperson were to venture into the reference room, he or she might mistake it for a three-ring circus. This madness, however, was cleverly orchestrated by the handful of people involved in getting initial access to the filings. All players were basically on the same page of the playbook as to what document and which filer to look for. For example, there were rumors in early 1987 that Piedmont Airlines, now a wholly-owned company of US Airways, was under attack by the well-known corporate raider Carl Icahn. Skip and the boys were up on the latest gossip and news, as they read the *Wall Street Journal, Investor's Business Daily,* and several other business publications each day before the market opened at 9:30 a.m. (EST). On this particular day, Carl Icahn made a filing on Piedmont Airlines, with the crux of the filing centering on the notion that Icahn was unsure whether he and his group would be able to obtain financing for the acquisition. This was huge information with potentially important implications. Skip and Phillip dissected the filing and were among the first to realize that financing the deal was in jeopardy.

Each of the five trial arbitrageurs had a designated printer that only received information disseminated by Skip's company. The information was delivered via satellite to a dish installed in each of the client's offices. The objective was that each client receive the information simultaneously, which was not an easy feat in the 1980s. Technology was still developing, and it was still the pre-Internet era. While Skip and Phillip were researching companies as possible distributors, Western Union was vying for their business. In his due diligence, Skip asked the voluptuous saleswoman if her clients would be able to receive their information simultaneously, and she said of course—one after the other. It turned out that Western Union possessed more beauty than brains; it seemed large, SAT-type words like "simultaneous" were foreign to them. The boys found a group who actually could distribute the information simultaneously via satellite, and so the ball began rolling. For all intents and purposes, the information was received within seconds of each other, which was good enough.

With respect to Carl Icahn and the Piedmont deal, one of the five trial clients called and asked Skip if he was sure that he and Phillip had read the document correctly, because not having financing in place could impact the price of Piedmont stock. An anxious Skip and Phillip quickly re-read the lengthy document and assured the arbitrageur, one of their largest clients, that they were sure the information was correct.

The trading day was over and Skip and Phillip were winding down operations when the phone rang. It was the same "arb" who had pressed them earlier about the Piedmont deal. Apprehensive, Skip took the call and listened intently. Because of the information the boys had sent out to this arb and their other clients concerning the Icahn financing, the price of Piedmont Airways went down almost six dollars per share. The arb had called to thank them; they shorted the stock based upon the boys' information and made nearly one million dollars on that transaction alone. The arb told Skip to sign them up as a client for life.

✝

Dr. Stanley Engel saw Skip soon upon his return from Europe. Skip had all but forgotten the initial consultation and was expecting the doctor to go over the test results, after which Skip would be on his merry way. The news from Dr. Engel was not good. What was supposed to be a routine exam with normal results was anything but. The nodule initially found in Skip's throat was a malignant thyroid tumor: the extent of its growth and damage had yet to be determined. Skip made the visit to Dr. Engel's alone and found himself wandering off into the clouds of confusion, trying to come to terms with the conversation at hand. "Did the doctor just tell me that I have cancer? This certainly can't be so. I'm only twenty-nine years old with my whole life before me," Skip thought to himself.

Thyroid cancer, an uncommon type of cancer, develops when abnormal cells begin to grow in one's thyroid gland. (The thyroid gland is shaped like a butterfly and is located in the front of your neck.) Most people who have it do very well because the cancer is usually found early and the treatments work well. After it is treated, thyroid cancer may come back, sometimes many years after treatment.

In Skip's case, a biopsy would be performed to determine which type of thyroid cancer he had, types that ranged from the benign papillary carcinoma to the more extreme anaplastic thyroid cancer, for the type of cancer cell found would dictate his course of treatment. As Skip quickly realized, it seemed that everything in the medical field took time: scheduling tests, the biopsy, and obtaining the results. The medical science field moved much more slowly than Skip's fast-paced world of stock trading. Waiting and patience were two characteristics that Skip would struggle with, especially when they revolved around health issues.

The biopsy was scheduled for a week from Tuesday. A week. That it could take that long to get something done was hard for Skip to believe. Except in extreme emergencies, it appeared the world of medical science trudged along at its own pace for whatever reasons. Waiting is the hardest part. During moments like these, deep thinking, faith, and prayer usually surface. Skip was young, full of Wall Street and personal charisma, and wasn't sure about dipping his feet into the pool of faith just yet. But those around him were. His family prayed and sent out messages to prayer groups and churches that the cancer would not be serious but curable, and probably anything else one would need a prayer for in such circumstances.

✝

The Lombardi Comprehensive Cancer Center at Georgetown University Hospital was a quick trip on the Metro. From the Foggy Bottom stop, it was a brief walk to the hospital. Skip was anticipating that his parents would pick him up after the biopsy procedure. After the usual laborious check-in and paperwork, Skip was greeted by a young nurse who took him back to a room where he would be prepped for the procedure.

The thyroid nodule was penetrated with a needle that removed material from the thyroid in an attempt to further diagnose the type of cancer with which they were dealing. The procedure was quick and relatively painless, and Skip was pleasantly surprised when it was over. The sample was whisked off to pathology where it would be examined and the results reported back to Dr. Engel, who would inform Skip of the results. Again, it was a waiting game. How long to get the results? Several days perhaps. While the majority of thyroid biopsies turn out to be papillary in nature, it was still possible to get the more serious type and all of the repercussions that go with it. Regardless of the type, surgery was in Skip's future. The thought of someone slitting his throat on purpose was enough to keep him up at night.

†

By the mid-1980s, the mergers and acquisitions business was in full swing. The small company with three founding members boasted a staff of over seventy-five employees and revenues in a realm beyond their wildest expectations. Skip and the others knew that there were basically two ways to make money with an entrepreneurial venture: either grow the business, utilize the cash flow, and distribute that money via dividends or by some other method to themselves and the employees or sell the business. Every company employee held stock in the firm—from Skip, Mark, and Phillip down to the secretaries and those who copied documents in the SEC reading room. It was a founding principle that people would work harder and become more motivated if they had a piece of the pie, regardless of its size. As the company grew, employees would be financial winners no matter what. More cash flow meant bigger bonuses and larger salaries along the way. It also meant that each share was worth more as the company grew; thus, if the company was sold at a later date, the share price for each employee would continually increase.

The original business model had the company being sold five years down the road, as opposed to taking cash out of the business along the way. Events in the timetable had occurred faster than the group expected. The company paid back its original investors, a board of directors made up of distinguished Washington businessmen, academicians from American University, and prominent local money managers. The plan was to pay the investors back within two years, and the firm accomplished just that. No longer flying under the radar, the company was known by virtually every player in the mergers and acquisitions arena on and off Wall Street. With growing attention and profitability came growing interest in acquiring the young start-up. Those most likely to be suitors were directly involved in the business themselves, or had an ancillary interest in news or merger information. From the inception to the sell, Dow Jones and Company appeared to be a natural collaborator as an acquiring partner, able to give the company both the value that it thought it deserved via its shares, and a business partnership that would benefit both organizations in the long run. Also in the running was the Bloomberg Company, founded by the now-famous mayor of New York City and former bond trader extraordinaire, Michael Bloomberg. Like Dow Jones, Bloomberg had a major presence in just about every location that Skip's company would like to pursue. Up to this point, Skip's claim to fame, or fifteen minutes of greatness, was having lunch with Michael Bloomberg to discuss, among other things, a possible business collaboration. Skip recalled Bloomberg's recommending a sushi restaurant near his office. Having used raw fish only as bait for larger fish, Skip responded with, "Of course, Mr. Bloomberg. I love sushi."

†

The results were in, and Dr. Engel immediately summoned Skip to his office to go over the findings. Skip mulled over the possibilities as he made his way along K Street to Dr. Engel's office, dissecting each possible outcome, both the positive and more deleterious. The results of the needle biopsy suggested that Skip had papillary carcinoma of the thyroid gland, the most benign of the several types of thyroid cancer, which, paradoxically, was good news for Skip. Still, surgery would be needed, and it was delicate terrain operating on that part of the body. Dr. Engel was one of the best in town, and Skip felt comfortable utilizing his expertise. The surgery was scheduled at George Washington Hospital the following week. In addition to the surgery, Skip would be placed on a thyroid hormone after the surgery since his would be almost totally removed. The thyroid hormone is used to treat hypothyroidism, a condition where the thyroid gland does not produce enough thyroid hormone, or it is given to those who've had their thyroid removed. Without this hormone, the body cannot function properly, resulting in poor growth, slow speech, lack of energy, weight gain, hair loss, dry or thick skin, and increased sensitivity to cold. Chemotherapy and radiation therapy are generally not treatment options at this level. Skip was anxious over the upcoming surgery, and again prayers were prayed for him. Yet, he appeared to find more comfort in the fact that Dr. Engel was the best surgeon in town. It was only a matter of time before Skip would revisit his derivation of faith.

A millionaire by thirty. The American dream. The house in the upscale Barnaby Woods neighborhood in northwest Washington, DC. The beautiful, young wife. Skip had it all, didn't he? The company was eventually sold to Dow Jones and Company for a multiple that made the three founders rich and most of the employees more money than they had ever expected. The deal was that Dow Jones would buy 80 percent of the company upfront and the remaining 20 percent a few years later. Skip's company needed to stay in tack and grow over those next few years to maximize the value of the remaining 20 percent. This is where "Greed is Good" and acrimony come into the picture. The months and years after the buyout were representative of Virgil's Hell, with Skip and Phillip crying out for help, but their efforts were of little avail. As with any business deal gone awry, the animosity led to a legal dispute over who gets what and how much. In the end, Mark came away with the lion's share, as perhaps he should since it was his initial conception. Skip and Phillip earned the right to receive the value of their 20 percent remaining stake. So ends the tale of the entrepreneurs. Anecdotally, upon moving into the house in northwest Washington, Skip would go to work wearing Bermuda shorts and a T-shirt, weather permitting. One of the next-door neighbors, a woman in her midforties, asked Ashley where Skip worked that allowed him to wear that kind of getup and afforded him the luxury of buying their current property. Ashley recounted the *Reader's Digest* version to the neighbor and, as she departed, the next-door neighbor asked Ashley when her parents were moving in. The mistake of putting

Ashley in the upscale Barnaby Woods neighborhood at twenty five years old would come back to haunt him.

✝

The thyroid surgery had gone well. Another perfect procedure by Dr. Engel. Although his recuperation would last several weeks, Skip was out of the hospital the next day, back at home on the coach with painkillers nursing his wounds. Then came the customary visits from friends, family, and coworkers, and while Skip enjoyed these visits, he really just wanted to relax and get better. The thyroid that was removed was kept frozen by the hospital for reasons not known to Skip. It would prove vital that the specimen was kept, for years later the frozen tissue would need to be reexamined.

Chapter 4

THE PROCESS BEGINS

✝

Maria would eventually remarry and move out from under the elder Celia's dwelling. It would take a strong and courageous woman to endure the continual onslaught of pain and suffering that had been and would be inflicted upon her and the family over time. Every family at some point will experience trials and tribulations. But for the Sibley family, tragedy would incessantly raise its ugly head.

Skip had just earned his liberal arts degree and was going to continue on to graduate school in business. Jacqueline, the younger sibling of two years, was beginning her second term in college when God regained the attention of the family. Jacqueline had become depressed and was under a psychiatrist's care for several psychotic episodes. The transcendence was not outwardly displayed by her character. Jacqueline, at least in her own tormented mind, did not fit into this natural world.

✝

It was time to find a doctor to help both Skip and Ashley progress. Skip did very little in this process, as he still suffered intense pain the majority of the time with his arm in a sling. Even though there were several major hospitals in the greater Charleston area, the number of oncologists was limited. Ashley had researched via the Internet and made calls to friends and others who had connections to oncologists in the area. Ashley finally scheduled an appointment for Skip to see Dr. Barker from the Palmetto Oncology Group. Dr. Barker was ten to fifteen years older than Skip, and the two hit it off immediately. Dr. Barker was a local Charlestonian who received his medical training at the Harvard of the South: Vanderbilt. His compassion and empathy were evident, and his voice indicated that he wanted nothing less than to heal Skip completely. Ashley, or a proxy, would need to accompany Skip as Skip could not drive. He also had difficulty remembering the gist of his office visits with Dr. Barker. As the doctor was working with minimal information from the emergency room in Abbeboro, he was basically starting from scratch. Dr. Barker was in practice with two other doctors who would take part in Skip's care.

Based upon Skip's medical history and his previous cancer of the thyroid, Dr. Barker surmised that the thyroid cancer had most likely metastasized to the bone in the arm. This frequently happened with papillary carcinoma of the thyroid gland. Obviously, the type of cancer must be determined before the treatment plan was created. Dr. Barker did the usual blood work and sent Skip on several other odysseys at Roper Hospital that Skip would become all too familiar with over the next months and years. Dr. Barker quickly ordered magnetic resonance imaging (MRI) of the relevant body parts that were likely to provide information such as the humeral area of the right arm and the lungs. A total body bone scan was also ordered to see if there was any distant metastasis to other parts of the body. A biopsy of the tumor would also be required—this being the true litmus test of determining what type of cancer Skip really had. All of these tests were needed to determine the point of origin and type of cancer so that a regimen of healing could commence.

Anyone who has ever had an MRI is familiar with that claustrophobic feeling that creeps up when one is inside the MRI machine. The MRI tube is essentially the size of one's body, with very little room at the top and sides. If one had an itch on his or her foot, for example, there is no way of scratching it. Skip had to practice mind over matter to push away itches and panic attacks while being scanned for sometimes up to half an hour. He also wore an herbal eye pack that contained a soothing element that would make the trip into the MRI more manageable. Often, one's body is injected with a dye or contrast, as it was with Skip, which enhances the MRI scan images. Used in about 20 percent of MRI cases, it is usually ordered for patients with cancer or for those who might have a tumor. The MRIs were no trip to Hollywood. Skip dreaded each one he endured, both initially and over the years that followed. The nurses would pipe music into the tube to make the experience as soothing as possible. Skip remembered once having an itch on his leg and starting to freak out that he couldn't scratch it. To gain some relief, he willed the itch up to his head so that he could rub his head against the side of the MRI tube. So many little insults along the road to healing.

A bone scan or PET scan (or both) can also be used to further diagnose a patient and was used in Skip's case. PET is a nuclear medicine technique that uses a camera to capture powerful images of the human body's function and reveals information on health and disease. Compounds normally existing in the body, like simple sugars, are labeled with radioactive tracers that emit signals and are injected into the body intravenously. The scanner records the signals that the tracer emits as it journeys through the body and as it collects in targeted organs. A powerful computer reassembles the signals into actual images that then show biological maps of normal organ function and failure of organ systems in disease.

The PET scan and bone scan, each performed on Skip, were both relatively benign and noninvasive. The scariest thing about the scan was waiting for the outcome or results, which never seem to be available right away. Skip had to wait on a call or pay a visit to Dr. Barker to glean the results.

A biopsy was performed at Roper Hospital to remove a portion of Skip's tumor so the pathologists could determine the kind of cancer. Unlike the thyroid biopsy, this was serious surgery. Skip was awake but anesthetized during the procedure that seemed to take a long time. The operating room visit, Skip's first since his thyroid incident, had all the warm fuzzies of a kick in the mouth. It was cold. Everyone wore masks, and no one was smiling. They had either switched to drinking decaf coffee or were very concerned about the procedure. Skip's guess would be the latter. The surgeon and pathologist were present to take the biopsied specimen to the lab right away to determine if the surgeon had removed enough tissue to get a reading. This process again seemed to drag on, but Skip knew that all involved were doing their best and were there for him. The pathologist determined the tissue sample was sufficient (barely), so they closed Skip up at that point. Again, the tumor was located in the upper or lateral part of Skip's right arm, which immediately went back into the sling, followed by another round of pain meds.

The major determinative tests had been done. It was now a waiting game.

✝

What went wrong? What went so terribly wrong in the body, mind, and spirit of Jacqueline? The psychiatrists determined that she was of no harm to herself or others, so she was released from the ward to the custody of her parents. Several weeks went by and Jacqueline showed no particularly troubling signs to Maria and Mack, Jacqueline's stepdad. Mack was a large man of few words and loved the children that he had inherited, Skip and Jacqueline, as well as his own young son Scott, who was birthed by Maria. Kind to a fault, he would do just about anything for anyone. A civil servant, he worked for the Social Security Administration for most of his working years. The family spent all of their lives living in the suburbs of Washington, DC.

Jacqueline was under constant supervision, and the family was instructed to notify the doctor immediately if her state of mind or condition worsened.

Scott Sibley—the handsome, teenage son of Maria and Mack—was at home during this time. Did he understand the nature of the situation with his sister?

The family station wagon had been running in the garage with the garage door closed as Maria and Mack pulled into the driveway. Although Jacqueline was obviously of age to drive, her meds prohibited her from going behind the wheel. Jackie, sweet and precious Jackie, why? As Mack quickly flung the garage door open, the first thing that hit him was the billowing fumes from the exhaust of the vehicle. Jackie lay in a fetal position under the exhaust pipe, lifeless. She had been inhaling lethal fumes from the exhaust pipe for an undetermined amount of time.

The house became a crime scene with the police, Emergency Medical Services, and every emergency vehicle in the area showing up to determine what took place. Jackie, sweet Jackie, was gone at the tender age of twenty-one. Her death was ruled a suicide and her body taken away to one of those cold places where bodies go before loved ones get to grieve over it. It is unimaginable, the emotions that Maria and Mack must have experienced. One of the suppositions in life is that parents are not supposed to bury their own children.

Where are you, Jacqueline? Doesn't the Catholic Church say that suicide is a sin that bans people from heaven? How could an omnipotent and empathetic God send sweet Jackie to hell? These were the questions that were whirl-winding through Skip's mind as he raced home from Gettysburg College. Skip, at this point in his young life, had never set foot in the college chapel, and the only time he found himself in church was at a family or friend's wedding. The grief that overcame the Sibleys would manifest differently in each of the surviving family members. Goodbye, Jackie.

†

The MRI of the humerus bone came back with predictable results. Skip's tumor had a mass the size of a walnut. The MRI confirmed what the x-rays had already indicated, that there was a mass of some kind in the upper right arm. What kind of mass had yet to be determined. The lungs showed negative on its MRI, a blessing for sure. Still, Skip was not sure how to interpret this first bit of news. A tumor mass had been confirmed, but whether it was benign or malignant and the nature of the beast was a mystery. Dr. Barker was still operating under the assumption that he was dealing with a thyroid tumor that had metastasized to the arm bone. It had been almost ten years since the thyroid cancer, at this point. However, the spread of malignant thyroid cells can take place many years from its onset. To Skip, x-rays were one thing; one could look at the image and basically see what was going on. Skip realized then why radiologists went to school for as long as they did and made the kind of money they made. Looking at MRIs was another matter. To Skip, the MRI looked like a ham that was being sliced horizontally, rendering it meaningless. Skip was the patient; he wasn't paid to read the MRIs. With MRIs in hand and pain ever present, Skip waited for the results of the bone scan.

Other than his visits with Dr. Barker, Skip perceived the medical field as very cold and detached. It wasn't like General Hospital, where the beautiful nurse came in at regular intervals to offer the patient a sponge bath. It was a stoical environment, one to which he was not accustomed. The reprieves and the sympathy came only during his visits to Dr. Barker's office, where he was cared for by the doctor and his nurse, Diane. Although the office was steps away from the hospital, it was worlds away in attitude and optimism. At this point, Skip was required to visit the doctor's office two to three times a week, but it was difficult getting downtown as Ashley worked and Skip could not drive himself. A combination of family and friends put together a schedule and got Skip to and from his appointments the best they could.

The bone scan results confirmed what the MRI had shown. The area in the proximal humerus was hot, or lit up, on the bone scan, meaning this was an area of interest to the doctors. It was the only place on the bone scan that presented a problem at this point. The radiologist did note in his report that a metal object of unknown origin was worn around the neck of the patient. Skip had forgotten to take off his St. Christopher's medal before the scan. Skip had recently started wearing it again; he had received it in high school. Skip wanted to be armed with as much ammunition as possible to fight the battles to come.

The biopsy results took a little longer as they were sent to several local pathologists in order to determine the type of cancer. This was the big kahuna in the process thus far. Presently, treatment was being led locally by Dr. Barker, and tests, scans, and so forth were, for the most part, being done at Roper Hospital. As it turned out, the specimen gathered during the biopsy was small, and the pathologists were having trouble determining its significance. It was Skip's understanding that a biopsy couldn't be performed twice, for reasons he was unsure of. Pathologists in Charleston, a relatively small city, didn't usually see rare diseases in any significant quantity. Nevertheless, the tissue sample from the biopsy was sent to a local pathology group. But weeks later, Skip was still waiting for what, at the time, would be the most important news in his life. Every day, either Skip or Ashley would call Dr. Barker's office to see if there was any news. The waiting game continued.

†

Things at home were hectic. How does one begin to describe the chaos that defined the daily lives of the Sibleys? For Skip, there was pain and more pain and endless trips to the doctor. During this pathological waiting game, Skip underwent a myriad of other tests and routines to either locate or rule out a body part that might be the cause of the tumor. Gastroenterologists checked for any warning signs in the digestive tract. The doctor told Skip he would perform both a colonoscopy and a gastronomic procedure whereby the scope would be placed down Skip's throat, to which Skip replied, "Do you mind sending the scope down my throat before you use it to look in my butt? I would hate to have it the other way around." Speaking of butts, Skip recalled, with a grin on his face, a recent incident when both Foster and Caroline were sick. Since Foster was just a baby, they had a thermometer just for him with the word "butt" written on it, because at that time it was the standard, most reliable way to get an accurate reading.

Well, one day Ashley is walking by the couch where she sees Caroline trying to take her own temperature. As Ashley moves closer to Caroline, she doesn't know whether to cry or laugh, as Caroline is propped on the couch with a thermometer sticking out of her mouth with the word "butt" written on it. It certainly set the tone for events in the near future.

✝

Finally, a call from Diane at Dr. Barker's office. The biopsy results were in and Dr. Barker had requested that Skip make an appointment to discuss the results. An appointment could not be worked in for two days, and Diane could not relay any information to Skip over the phone. Patience. Torture. Anxiety. Fear. These were just a few of the emotions that plagued Skip.

For what credit is it if, when you are beaten for your faults, you take it patiently? But, when you do good and suffer, if you take it patiently, this is commendable before God.

1 Peter 2:20

Dr. Barker gave Skip the most likely scenario: the thyroid tumor had metastasized to the bone in the arm. It was not a great scenario, but at least it could be treated.

The initial pathology was complete. It confirmed Dr. Barker's speculations that the metastasis had come from the thyroid. Skip thought that the whole thyroid situation was taken care of years ago, but here it was again, back in a distant form and location. With results in hand, it was time to go to work. Another test would be performed to validate the pathological findings. Skip was admitted to Roper for several days and taken off his thyroid medicine to force his body into a hypothyroid state. Test after test and scan after scan, the process seemed endless, and at times hopeless. One cannot live without the thyroid, that small and seemingly inconsequential gland in the throat. The major advance in thyroid cancer treatment over the last decade had been the ability to calculate the absorbed radiation dose in recurrent or metastatic tumors that concentrate radioiodine. Skip was given a radioactive iodine solution that would, in some way, determine thyroid involvement. He was isolated in a room at the hospital for several days in order for the findings to be collected, which gave him time to think. The usual questions surfaced: Why me? What next? The children? Will I die? The stress was internalized for the most part as there appeared to be some hope. The isotopic iodine was another link in the ongoing mystery, but it kept the path of thyroid metastases open.

Believing that he was dealing with metastatic thyroid cancer, Dr. Barker began aggressive radiation therapy to Skip's right arm. At such high does, radiation could have deleterious, long-term consequences, but it seemed that every short-term treatment had side effects that could be detrimental. However, when one is told one has cancer, one does whatever it takes to get rid of it, so was the opinion of Skip. The radiation therapy was every day for two months. The radiologist made a certain guard or screen for Skip to direct the radiation to only the part of the body where the tumor is located. Skip would lie on a table each day while the nurses prepared the radiation machine for its killing duties. Although science has advanced at an incredible pace, with radiation treatment, it is impossible to target only the tumor cells, so healthy cells are damaged along the way. One's body can endure only so much radiation in a lifetime, which is why during dental or other x-rays, a lead shield is placed across nonassociative body parts in order to prevent additional radiation from being absorbed into the body. The radiation was again noninvasive; however, it did zap Skip's energy levels and left burn marks where the radiation hit the body. Skip didn't know it at the time, but high doses of radiation in his case were likely to cause additional sarcomas in the future. How far in the future was anyone's guess.

Chapter 5

OPTIONS

†

Ashley was diligent with her research on the disease. On the Internet she found an array of statistics, studies, and options available to cancer patients. One recurring theme kept coming back to her and Skip. Should they ask for a second opinion? Most of the research Ashley had uncovered suggested getting not only a second and third opinion, but also consulting one of the country's major cancer treatment centers. Charleston had a number of adequate medical facilities. However, having cancer and birthing babies were two totally different uses of a hospital and its personnel. The nearest major cancer center to Charleston was in Durham, North Carolina, at the Duke University Hospital Center. It was well-known and well-respected for its Cancer Clinic. Ashley and Skip decided to take a trip to Duke, although it had never been suggested by Dr. Barker or anyone locally at Roper or any other facility the Sibleys had visited.

At first glance, the Duke Clinic was one of the most depressing places Skip had ever seen. A massive room was filled with patients and their families or advocates, and for them this was their hope. "I want to leave immediately," said Skip, as he perused the vacuous crowd. The place was full of wheelchairs, crutches, baldness, and people getting sick to their stomachs. A ghostly pale covered the patients' faces. While this was ostensibly a place of hope and cure, one could see only pain and suffering in the eyes of the burdened. Despair hung in the air as the fall dew on the vine. There must have been hundreds of people there waiting their turn to see the doctor of the day. Skip wondered how they could cycle through this many people in a day. The staff must have been large and expedient.

The one advantage of coming to a place like Duke was that by being a major cancer center, what is rare in Charleston is much less so at Duke. The local pathologist in Charleston may see one or two samples like Skip's a year, if that, whereas the pathologists at Duke see this kind of cancer many times a year. The wait was several hours, but that was to be expected. Other than wearing a sling on his right arm, Skip, even in the shape he was in, looked like Robert Redford compared to those other waiting room patients—at least on this visit.

✝

Was there any place to run and hide? Could he just snap his fingers and make it all go away? Surely, this was a dream, and he would awaken soon. At the end of the day, Skip had these same thoughts and emotions. Each night at regular intervals, he would wake in a sweat, realizing that it wasn't a dream at all. Reality sunk in once again as he came to terms with the dimensions of his suffering. Emotions ran the gamut of the grief cycle almost daily. Life as normal continued around him while he toiled with his misery. Does life miss a beat when you are gone? Does the world stop on a dime to offer its condolences? The universe is so vast and never ending, and death and a never ending world continued to present itself to him. Our sovereign God most certainly sees the plan. Family and close friends had gone on before him, and the world hadn't blinked as far as he could tell. Would this be true of his death if it occurred?

It's 4:30 a.m. on a Tuesday
It doesn't get much worse than this
In beds in little rooms in buildings in the middle
Of these lives which are completely meaningless
Help me stay awake, I'm falling...
Adam Duritz

✝

"Malcolm Sibley," said the voice from behind the desk. It was finally Skip's time. The chaos in the waiting area became a well-orchestrated sonata behind closed curtains. Dr. Laurie and his well-mentored minions, as Duke was a teaching hospital, all flaunted over to Skip and Ashley. The doctor then presented Skip's case back to him in remarkable detail. Skip had presumed that after walking in from the waiting room, the doctor would have no notion of his case, and it would take time to research, read, and study Skip's situation. Nothing could be farther from the truth. Dr. Laurie exuded confidence. He was familiar not only with Skip's case, but also with the possible types of cancer. The biggest piece of any cancer puzzle is the pathology. Dr. Laurie had studied the information sent to him from Dr. Barker via Diane that suggested metastatic thyroid cancer. As was hoped and expected, Dr. Laurie suggested that Duke take the lead on their case.

The downside? More delays. Dr. Laurie needed the biopsied tissue sample so the pathologists at Duke could make their own determination. One of Dr. Laurie's staff would make the arrangements, and upon finding the pathological results, they would meet again to discuss the findings.

While nothing was really gained on the trip to Duke, Skip and Ashley felt confident in their decision to share Skip's case with as many eyes as possible. The five-hour ride back to Charleston was uneventful as Ashley drove and Skip rested and pondered his next visit to Dr. Laurie.

✝

The trip to Duke had comforted Skip, but the uncertainty still lingered. Uncertainty in any realm can cause havoc. The stock market wants information. The economy and politics are intertwined in the need to push out information to the public. Ambiguity in the form of medical diagnosis is particularly tough on the soul. You know the world does not revolve around you or your particular circumstances, and you don't really want it to anyway. Hope is truly eternal, but the anonymous eats around the edges of optimism, leaving you struggling within yourself.

> For whatever things were written before were written for our learning,
> that we through the patience and comfort of the Scriptures
> might have hope.
> Romans 15:4

Did Ashley have the same feelings of hope and healing? They didn't talk about it. Ashley was less metaphysical at this point and more concerned with the pragmatic documentation that was unfolding before them. She would sit tight until the doctors at Duke revealed their own pathological findings. The waiting and the uncertainty did not seem to affect Ashley. She was stoic in one sense, but she had so much going on around her with work, children—especially a new son—and the patient. It was so overwhelming that she couldn't focus solely on any one aspect; it would drive her mad. But Skip could only speculate at this point.

✝

Back in Bay Club and Charleston, the world had not changed; life and its struggles were still confronting the Sibleys. The family was attempting to get back on a schedule that would help facilitate the day-to-day chores. Skip was again heading down to the hospital for his daily dose of radiation. Ashley was continuing to work. At this time, it was necessary to put Foster in day care, since family was not close enough to help. Ashley made the arrangements, but it broke Skip's heart that he was not able to care for his newborn son, a guilt that didn't help an already vulnerable Skip. As he waited on the radiation table or in the waiting room, he wondered what little Foster was doing at the time. Ashley was the modern woman who,

Skip believed, would have put Foster in day care even if Skip hadn't been sick. Skip was, call it old-fashioned, of the mind-set that if you are going to have a child, you need to be able to raise it yourself. Skip was no misogynist, but he chastised women who left their newborns with strangers. Certain situations, like their own, relied upon the care that was given by the day care facilities. Skip knew that the majority of children being dropped off at day care each day had mothers who needed to work, not just to help with household expenses, but to buy houses and cars that they really didn't need and couldn't afford. "Who am I to judge?" thought Skip. People have their priorities, and there is usually no changing them. It seemed to Skip that sacrifices should be made so that one of the parents could stay home to raise their child. This often is not possible, with the myriad of single mothers in the world, and the need for extra income from those fortunate enough to have a nuclear family. Women work hard, and have to juggle many balls in order to make it through the day. Times have changed.

Shortly after Caroline was born and the family had moved south to Charleston, Skip took some time off after selling the mergers and acquisitions business and spent a year at home with their newborn Caroline. If all men had an opportunity to play Mr. Mom, for any extended period, there would be a newfound respect for child rearing in this country. After coming off one of the most stressful career paths of Wall Street mergers and acquisitions, Skip was now thrust into his new at-home career, which would be every bit the challenge of the financial world. Where to begin? At this point in time, not many men stayed home with their children while the female held down a full-time job. What Skip remembers most from this period is that with child in tote, he rarely had a moment to himself. Grabbing a meal, taking a shower, or even going to the bathroom had to be planned and coordinated around the baby's schedule. The days seemed endless: up early and down late with chaos ensuing in between. The highlight of Skip's day would be his long afternoon nap on the couch, when Caroline would fall asleep on Skip for sometimes hours at a time. Skip wasn't sure where Caroline fell on the difficult-baby scale or whether she was a high-maintenance baby. His guess was that she was higher maintenance than most. Ashley would agree with this, as they waited some five years before having Foster. Caroline and her self-determination kept pushing the idea of a second child farther and farther into the future.

The days of taking care of Caroline, as difficult as they were, were his relatively carefree days. Back then, what was thought to be happiness came more frequently, and life moved forward without much difficulty. Indeed, Skip's time at home with Caroline was the best time, the closest to eternal bliss, or joy, that Skip had known. What could be better than spending moments that will last a lifetime with your new daughter?

Skip's visions of diapers, baby bottles, and strolls in the park seemed distant, yet ever present.

The routine, if one could call it that, was becoming more instinctual for both father and daughter. The pinnacle of each day was when Ashley came walking through the door, whereby Caroline was thrust upon her by Skip, and Caroline would smile and giggle at seeing Momma after a long day's absence. These days progressed, and the calendar pages turned ever so slowly.

✝

Margaret Brown from next door stopped by to see how things were going. Ashley filled her in on the latest news about Skip that would soon make its way around Bay Club. Margaret had mentioned something unusual, which had piqued Ashley's interest. Margaret had told Ashley about a young man named Nick who did yard work and other handyman jobs around the house for Margaret. In conversation, Margaret mentioned Skip and his condition to Nick, who immediately felt a bond with Skip, although the two had never met. Nick was a one-time Naval cadet at Annapolis, but was discharged for reasons unknown. He was a pleasant fellow with long hair and a beard, and he always looked dirty, perhaps because of his constant toiling in the yard. Nick was what one might call an evangelical Christian, although he did not attend any particular church. Nick would spend time talking to folks at the homeless shelter, or he would sit at Hardee's or Wendy's for hours preaching the Word and buying someone down on his luck a burger or sandwich. Nick was always in prayer and seemed to be at peace with himself, although there were underlying currents that suggested Nick was not right.

Nick had asked Margaret if he and a friend could come over to Ashley and Skip's house to pray for Skip and talk a little. Ashley asked Skip what he wanted to do. Skip had not been to church for a while and needed all the help he could get during his time of need, so he told Ashley to set it up with Margaret to have the guys over.

Nick, Ed, and Steve knocked on the door on a Tuesday night at Skip and Ashley's house. Ed was the eldest of the three, slightly older than Skip, and had a familiar New York accent. Steve was the most soft spoken of the three. Skip would find out later that Steve had HIV and was suffering in his own way. All three were outspoken Christians and believed in the healing powers of God through Jesus.

> But a certain Samaritan, as he journeyed, came where he was
> And when he saw him, he had compassion.
> So he went to him and bandaged his wounds, pouring on oil and wine;
> and he set him upon his own animal, brought him to an inn,
> and took care of him.
> Luke 10:33-34

At first Skip wasn't sure what to make of the three "wise men" who had gathered at his home that evening. Why had they come to see him? Why was his story so compelling? What innate kindness caused these men to venture over to a stranger's house to wish him well and to pray for his healing? Nick, you see, believed he heard the Word of God, not just in this instance, but throughout his everyday life. While some may consider this a blessing, Nick was full of the Holy Spirit, but was being tortured at the same time. It is said that those who are closest to God are most often attacked by the devil. Nick was brilliant, but he possessed a tortured soul. Nick also heard voices but at times could not distinguish the Godly from the demonic. Just as Jesus was tempted by Satan, so it appeared Nick was fighting a similar battle. The voices became too alarming, so Nick was forced to seek shelter for his own protection and the protection of others.

That night, Nick, Ed, and Steve prayed over Skip in a spirit-filled way that Skip had never felt. Ed brought a small canister of grape juice and a few pieces of bread and led a communion for those present. Nick brought with him a jar of olive oil and rubbed it gently on the cancerous part of Skip's arm, all while saying prayers of healing and laying on of hands and appearing to act as a conduit of God's word through the Holy Spirit. Ashley was vacant for the majority of the visit, while Skip was stunned at the spiritual orchestration of it all. Skip thanked them appreciably before they left, and all vowed to meet again in the near future.

Skip never saw Steve again but often wondered how he was doing with his HIV. Nick no longer worked next door at Margaret's house, so Skip didn't have any connection to his whereabouts, except through Ed who, for a while, was stopping by on a regular basis to see Skip and to offer him support both biblically and physically, as Ed was in the business of selling vitamins and supplements, all of which was new to Skip.

At first Skip didn't know what to make of this newfound evangelism, but it was clear that a pilot light was lit inside of him. Skip was taken back by it all. The pain and suffering. The upbringing in the Catholic Church and sin. The evangelical Christian message of hope and healing. What road was this leading down? Skip was just a neophyte and not ready for the full- blown version of Christianity, even though he allegedly practiced it his entire life. Like Nick, Skip was battling his own demons. In an internal system that was already overloaded, it would take time to process this new spirituality and maybe even incorporate the faith into his lifestyle. Skip believed in God, as did 90 percent of Americans, but he felt a small sanguine tugging that was in the right direction. Only time would tell.

Chapter 6

THE VERDICT

†

Back to Charleston once more. Ashley set up an appointment for Skip with Dr. Barker to review their meeting with the doctors at Duke. While Dr. Barker would get the notes from Dr. Laurie, Ashley thought it best that they meet in person to discuss the trip to Durham. Presently, the diagnosis was metastatic thyroid cancer that had spread to the humerus bone in Skip's right arm. Skip was roughly halfway through the radiation treatments, but he had no idea if he was doing well or if the treatments were working. Getting information out of anyone in the medical establishment was like pulling teeth, which only added to Skip's anxiety and deteriorating mental health. The dichotomy of the radiation treatment confused Skip. On one hand, it had the ability to shrink the tumor and perhaps kill it entirely. On the other hand, such high doses of radiation were not good for his body. It was as if a house was on fire and the only solution was to hose out the entire inside of the building. But he had chosen the short-term benefits over the longer-term implications.

†

It would take time, but behind the scenes at Duke the pathological movement had begun—a difficult case, even for a major cancer center like Duke. The pathology department at Duke was suspect from the beginning of the initial diagnosis in Charleston. The idea that metastatic thyroid cancer would come back some ten years later was possible, but not probable. Skip had a college friend whose father was a medical pathologist, and Skip thought he might be able to give him some insight. But, as Skip expected, it was impossible to tell anything without first looking at the cell samples. What he did learn, however, was that diagnosing something this rare was as much an art as it was a science. There are no cells with flags waving from them suggesting that they are this or that type of cancer.

And all this science I don't understand
it's just my job five days a week
a rocket man, a rocket man.
Elton John

The waiting was terminal. Each day Skip would awake from his silent nightmare and wonder why no decision had been made. Weren't they just looking at cells under a microscope? The complexity was beyond the comprehension of the still drug-induced patient. Finally, a call from Dr. Barker's office regarding the Duke pathology. Answers, finally.

†

One can only imagine the daily routine at the Sibley household. They say the caregiver is often under as much stress as those they care for. Ashley was up most of the night with newborn Foster. Skip was worthless to help, due to the arm, radiation, and the medication. With little to no sleep, Ashley arose to get Caroline ready for school and herself ready for work.

Caroline and Trovo would walk to the corner to await the bus that would whisk her off to kindergarten at Whitesides Elementary School. Ashley would finish getting ready before dropping Foster off at day care before her hour-long commute to work each way. Skip was home and would wake up to an empty house. Occasionally, a neighbor or someone from the church would come over to help him with food and getting to and from his radiation treatments. Life was hard and getting harder. Foster was a good baby, but a baby nonetheless. He demanded constant attention. So, day care provided a reprieve during the working hours. Ashley would fight the corporate grind and, at the end of her work day, begin her hour-long commute back to Bay Club. She loved seeing the kids, but she was so exhausted that it was difficult to spend any real quality time with them. How long could this continue? All involved were weary and weak. The full leap of faith had not yet occurred for Ashley or Skip. Each day took on a new meaning. No, they were not living in cardboard boxes in Quito, Ecuador, but all misery is relative to that of the beholder. The once-comfortable, marsh-front home in Bay Club no longer seemed to matter. No one had the strength, energy, or time to enjoy any of the comforts of home.

✝

Several weeks had passed since the visit to Duke. News that the results were ready was music to the ears of Skip and Ashley. In hindsight, it must have taken a while to get the actual tissue sample to Duke, and then additional time to analyze the material. Based upon the initial pathology, Dr. Barker's beliefs, and the visit to Duke, Skip thought the thyroid cancer would be confirmed, and he would finish up his radiation treatment and life would go on.

Dr. Barker painted the script like something from *Alice in Wonderland*. It was all upside down and backwards. Surely, there was a mistake. The expression on Dr. Barker's face suggested that he was deadly serious, and he truly regretted conveying the news. You see, it wasn't metastatic thyroid cancer at all; it was a cancer that originated in the bone, a sarcoma, a much, much more serious situation. This changed everything. Skip had that sinking feeling in his stomach again, the one that you get at the top of a roller coaster as it begins its descent. Untethered from reality once again, he met denial and disbelief. Ashley took control and wanted the name and number of the doctor who studied the tissue sample. She wanted to see more than a couple of sentences typed on a report on a cold piece of paper. It was difficult to get a hold of the doctor directly. In fact, it took much effort, as does everything as a medical patient or advocate. Finally her call was put through. She would not like what she was about to hear.

✝

Skip was doing his best to hold it together based on the new pathological diagnosis from Duke. His immediate intention was to chastise the folks in Charleston who made the original incorrect call. Or was it incorrect? Not only did Duke see the tissue sample, but the sample was also sent to the Mayo Clinic and Johns Hopkins for further analysis. In time, each pathologist came to the same conclusion. This was not metastatic thyroid cancer, but a bone sarcoma, Ewing's sarcoma to be exact. The early twentieth century physician James Ewing was the eponym of the tumor type. He was a professor and medical doctor at Cornell University.

Skip was skittering through the denial portion of the grief cycle. It was all coming at him now so fast and negative. What to do? Where to turn? Skip had an epiphany that he would contact the pathologist at Duke himself to hear firsthand whether this news was all correct. But picking up the phone was like walking into a haunted house. Fear was in all places. Palms were watering like Niagara Falls. Pick up the phone, he kept saying. Just make the call. Anxiety had given him partial paralysis. He picked up the phone and, after being transferred several times, the doctor of pathology was on the other end of the line. He seemed a nice enough gentleman who offered Skip the limited time and information that he had. He began by explaining how difficult it was to get an accurate reading due to the small tissue sample that was taken during the biopsy. While the doctor was speaking, Skip was doing his best to hold it together emotionally. Again, it was like a surreal, out-of-body experience. Skip was having this conversation, but he couldn't process it. The doctor spoke matter-of-factly, as if he were speaking to a colleague rather than a patient he has never met. In fact, most pathologists never speak to patients directly.

The news was stunning. By all accounts and confirmations of the other pathologists, the agreement was that they were dealing with the PNET/Ewing's type of tumor and not the thyroid tumor. Skip, barely able to speak, thanked the doctor for his time. The doctor displayed a modicum of empathy, perhaps not really realizing the weight of the message he was delivering. Skip hung up the phone, genuflected, and began to cry.

†

Ashley returned home from work that evening to find Skip lying on the floor of the bedroom in a fetal position. Ashley had contacted the pathologist herself and had an idea of what was going on. Skip told her the news, and they both hugged and cried. Ashley was devastated because she knew what the sarcomas were and what the life expectancy was as a result. Ashley left Skip momentarily to tend to Foster and Caroline and prepare something to eat and shut the bedroom door on her way out. Suddenly Skip felt an overwhelming yearning to bend to his knees and pray. It was difficult to tell whether Skip was experiencing loqutions from God or just wanted to be imparted with good news. In the midst of just receiving the distressing results, Skip felt a calmness and peace flowing through his body. His prayers were sophomoric at best, with requests for healing and to remain on Earth long enough to see his children grow. Skip was praying earnestly, as the tears rolled off his checks, for perhaps the first time in his pleadings with the Father. Little did he know that God was listening and that the auditory hallucinations were truly from the Holy Spirit. Later, this would become clear.

†

After learning the latest news, time was of the essence. Skip and Ashley packed the car one more time for another trip to Duke University Hospital. Skip's parents were there to watch the kids, which relieved some of Ashley's worry. During this whole waiting game of "discover the diagnosis," Skip remained with arm in sling and little ability to do anything.

Skip and Ashley would stay with their friends, the Claytons, who had three children and lived in Chapel Hill, each time they went to Duke. Conrad Clayton went to graduate school with Skip and was one of his roommates at American University. Now a successful entrepreneur in the Research Triangle area, Conrad created a software firm that would eventually be sold to a larger firm. His wife Peggy was one of the kindest people and would do just about anything to make her guests feel comfortable. Ashley and Peggy actually went to high school together in Greenwood, South Carolina. Peggy had her task cut out for her when the Sibleys arrived. This was a sad trip that was difficult for Skip. He wanted to interact with his friends but was unable to. All he could think of was their beautiful family and how he envied them. Skip was looking for normalcy, and the Claytons seemed to have just that. They had their health and their healthy lives. Skip knew that everyone had their baggage, but again it was all relative. Skip wanted assurances that he would be there for his children's high school graduation, their wedding, and so forth. As he looked at the Claytons, he thought about what he might miss out on in life—not so much his own life, but seeing his family grow.

†

They had a 9:00 a.m. appointment at the clinic, so Skip and Ashley were up and out of the Claytons' house early, driving the short distance from Chapel Hill to Durham. The Claytons actually lived right off the campus of North Carolina at Chapel Hill in a pristine location. The ride from one campus to another was about eight miles. The Duke campus was equally breathtaking in its architecture and charm, although it was full of negative connotations in Skip's mind, undermining the dramatic campus experience. They parked the Toyota Camry in the usual spot in the parking garage. Skip and Ashley were always carrying the latest x-rays, scans, and documentation from Dr. Barker in Charleston. They checked in at the reception area and took a seat in the cavernous waiting area.

An hour and fifteen minutes later, it was finally their turn. Again, they were directed to one of the offices of the clinic where the doctor would be there to see them shortly. This time, the meeting between patient and doctor was much more sobering. The doctor was cordial but firm in his analysis of the diagnosis. A basic physical was done with special attention given to the right arm. The doctor explained the pathological results and the overall picture of the Ewing's sarcoma. Both Skip and Ashley were determined, as are many cancer patients, to do whatever it takes and receive medically whatever is available to them to beat the disease. One thing that resonated with Skip was the treatment program outlined by the doctor. The doctor kept using the term "aggressive treatment" when referring to Skip's chemotherapy program. The doctor also mentioned the frequency and duration of the treatments, which at the time didn't mean much to Skip. But he would come to understand the meaning very quickly once the chemo began. The chemotherapy protocol was developed at St. Jude's Children's Hospital. The primary recipients of this type of cancer ranged in age from ten to twenty years old, which is why the treatment was developed at a children's hospital. St. Jude's is a wonderful facility responsible for groundbreaking research in many of the childhood cancers. Prior to St. Jude's developing the radiation, chemotherapy, and surgery protocol for Ewing's sarcomas, the mortality rate was approximately 85 percent for those diagnosed with the disease. All of these innovations had taken place in the last ten years or so.

In addition to the chemotherapy regimen, the doctors at Duke wanted that tumor out of Skip's arm and recommended surgery. The orthopedic oncologists at Duke wanted to use a cadaver humerus to replace the cancerous one in Skip's body. Right away, both Skip and Ashley withdrew when they heard the idea of using a dead person's bone in Skip's arm. Not only was the thought unappealing, but the doctors informed Skip that the rejection rate of the new bone was very high, and the chances of a major infection were also present. If this was the best alternative that Duke's surgeons could offer, Skip knew he was in a world of trouble. Skip had some time to make up his mind on the surgery because that would take place after the radiation was complete and the chemotherapy course was done. The chemotherapy routine was scheduled to last over a year, which, in terms of chemotherapy, is super aggressive.

Skip and Ashley said goodbye for now to the Claytons and headed homeward to Charleston. This time the conversation was livelier, as they had much to determine in the imminent future. Neither had a clue as to what the chemo would behold, but the idea of using a cadaver bone as a replacement didn't sit well with either of them.

✝

Dr. Barker had read the report from Duke and was to administer the chemotherapy to Skip throughout its course. Skip recalled Dr. Barker calling it "the beginning of the journey," something Skip would come to realize on his own. The St. Jude's chemotherapy would be long and harsh. The severity of the treatment required that Skip be an in-patient at the hospital for the chemo regimens. One regimen meant a week's stay, and then several weeks to regain strength and blood cells. After that, it was another four-or five-day hospital regimen with a different protocol of chemo drugs.

Hell is often thought of in the abstract, as a place where one might go after death. Some describe hell as being separated from God for eternity. Modern understandings of hell often depict it abstractly, as a state of loss rather than as fiery torture underground. Anyone who has ever undergone chemotherapy will tell you that there is a hell on Earth.

The first visit to Roper Hospital to start the chemo treatment was just as Skip expected. "It took time to get his room and the chemo going. The waiting truly was the hardest part. Skip and Ashley got to the hospital around 9:00 a.m. and were probably not admitted to their room until sometime after noon, with the chemotherapy nowhere in sight.

Ashley had spoken to the pharmacist at the hospital who said it was an unusual prescription, and so it took a little more time to locate and assemble. "More warm fuzzies about being the guinea pig for this protocol at the hospital," thought Skip. Before his admittance to the hospital several weeks prior, Skip had a surgical procedure that placed a so-called "life port" into the upper left side of his chest, which would facilitate the administering of the chemo drugs. Instead of having to find a vein each time a drug was administered, the nurse just inserted the needle into the life port, which was already connected to a major vein or artery. That life port, as Skip would realize, was a life saver.

It was finally time. The brew had been concocted, and it was time to be administered. Skip was anxious, as one could imagine, having to undergo his first chemotherapy session. He was dressed in a hospital gown and lay in bed as the first of the drugs was inserted into the life port. Ashley was there for support, although there was little that she could do, for this was the beginning of a long and arduous road for the two of them. It was about supper time, so Ashley said good-bye and returned to Bay Club to perform the usual household tasks and to care for the kids. Skip would be in the hospital on this initial visit for seven days, with an IV of poison constantly flowing into his system. Alone and uncomfortable, Skip started to feel the effects of the drugs. The nurses did their best to give their patients anti-nausea drugs but, in Skip's case, they only seemed to take the edge off. A wave of anxiety came over Skip, which caused him to get out of the bed and pace the floor. He felt as if he were coming out of his skin. Skip thought this was just par for the course, so he lived with this intense panic for the first several days, not wanting to complain or be a nuisance to the nursing staff.

The cafeteria staff brought food, but it was almost impossible to hold anything down; besides, Skip had no appetite. Finally, he reached his initial breaking point and summoned the nurses to help with his anxiety and pain. In tears and grief, Skip tried to explain his feelings to the nurse in order that she might help him. As a result, Dr. Barker ordered a strong dose of sedatives that would help calm Skip. They worked to a large degree. A year of this treatment had just begun; this fact consumed his thoughts. And he had fallen down on day one. Skip now understood what the doctors meant by aggressive therapy. Chemotherapy truly was hell on earth.

Chapter 7

LAYING ON OF HANDS

†

When he regained consciousness, Skip was gently helped to his feet by those who surrounded him. Weary and unsure of what had just happened, Skip slowly rose from his prone position to one of sitting upright. A clarity and peacefulness pervaded his mind and body. What just happened? Skip and David Gorham earlier that day had decided to go to Christ Church for a healing ceremony and a laying on of hands ritual. Neither Skip nor David knew for sure what to expect; would it be some kind of hocus pocus and snake oil, or possibly a legitimate visit from the Holy Spirit?

Laying on of hands is a ritual that has taken place in the many sects of Christianity, from Eastern Christianity to Catharism, Roman Catholicism, and more. The ritual is used as both a symbolic and formal method of invoking the Holy Spirit to heal those in need. The authority in the Christian church dates back to the Old Testament with blessings anointed to Isaac laying healing hands on Jacob, and a myriad of New Testament healings from not only Jesus but the apostles as well. The power of such healing comes from God, with Jesus and the apostles acting as conduits of such power. The apostles often invoked the name of Jesus and the Holy Spirit when performing their healing miracles.

Skip and David attended the Wednesday night service at Christ Church somewhat skeptical themselves, for it was the first time either had ventured into such a situation. David was Southern Baptist and Skip Catholic by baptism, but more nondenominational Christian now. Many churches offered healing services regardless of sect, especially the new and proliferating super nondenominational churches. They entered the church that was set in a contemporary style with music being played by a small band in the front of the chapel. Skip was better accustomed to the nontraditional style of worship, as that was the type of service that his family frequented on Sundays or an occasional Saturday night. David, on the other hand, attended a more traditional Baptist celebration with long-established hymns and no raising of the hands in worship and praise. The show tonight, however, was all about nontradition and the raising of hands and singing to the modern Christian music that dominated the contemporary worship service. They took a seat in the rear of the pews and watched and took part in the service. Some fifty people were there that evening, quite a crowd for a Wednesday night, David had thought. The idea to attend was David's. Although David suffered from a congenital heart disease, he, too, was looking for healing; but he was mainly interested in getting hands laid on Skip in his current battle with cancer. The service was pleasant, and both enjoyed the praise and worship that was offered. The laying on of hands was apparently the epilogue to the service, when those desiring a healing hand were asked to come to the front of the chapel while other parishioners filtered out. Skip and David hesitantly ventured toward the front to greet a dozen or so individuals who would lead them through the ritual. A nervousness and ill feeling came over Skip as he stood in the middle of a circle, surrounded by about six people. David was in a similar situation a few yards away. Skip heard the verbal praying and chanting, some perhaps in tongue, and felt the traditional hands being laid on his right arm at the site of the cancer. It is hard to determine how long this went on, but it was probably about five minutes. Skip was slowly moving toward a more tranquil state, with fatigue coming upon him. Peace. He definitely felt a sense of peace throughout the ritual. The last thing Skip remembered was a man's hand on his head, pushing Skip backwards ever so slightly. Skip had fallen backwards into the arms of the others who had gathered around him. David was also on his back on the ground when Skip looked in his direction. Both Skip and David arose. The power of the laying on of the hands had forced each of them to lose their balance and temporary consciousness and fall to the ground below. What had just happened? Did they really lose consciousness or was it a figment of their imagination? Did the power of the Holy Spirit conduct itself through these individuals tonight, as it had done in the days of the Old and New Testament? Only time would tell. Skip's experience was like nothing else he had ever encountered. Is it possible that these modern-day apostles were capable of performing the same healing functions as Peter and Paul in circa AD 5–10? Again, only time would tell.

✝

The chemotherapy dominated Skip's life. There were reprieves, for which he was grateful. Still, the majority of the early chemo days were spent on 5 South at Roper Hospital. Second only to the doom and gloom of the Duke Clinic, 5 South was generally a place where patients went before hospice, their last steps to the pearly gates. It was primarily a chemotherapy and cancer floor, but it also treated other patients with diseases like sickle-cell anemia and other blood disorders. Skip was on the St. Jude's protocol for bone cancer, which made him a regular to the floor. The routine was one week in the hospital and then two weeks at home to recover, and then back to the hospital for another round of weekly treatment. This would go on for a year or more. Dread, fear, panic, and all the usual lows that one might feel were felt by Skip on each visit to 5 South. When Ashley or whomever was taking him down for his treatment, he wondered about smaller things—the people and the traffic that surrounded them, for example. Where were they going? It was just another normal day in their lives. Going to work, running errands, taking the kids to school. Not many were heading to 5 South for a week of chemo.

Skip became friendly with most of the nursing staff and the others who worked on the floor, and he was visited daily by one of the doctors on duty, who would ask him how things were going. There were three doctors on staff at the Palmetto Oncology Group, the oncology associates that were assisting Skip. Dr. Barker was Skip's main doctor. A local Charlestonian with a degree from Vanderbilt, he saw Skip on a regular basis, both in the hospital and at the medical associate's office. Dr. Elizabeth Nicole was an associate of Dr. Barker who would visit Skip in the hospital on her rounds. Middle-aged with flowing blond-gray hair, she always brightened the hospital room when she came to check on Skip. Dr. Nicole also had a very positive outlook on life and survival that was so very important to patients on 5 South. The third doctor in the trio was Jim Cutter, who also visited Skip while making his rounds at Roper Hospital. Younger and much more pragmatic, he was mostly business on his visits. He and Skip would occasionally talk about cancer and the ability to cure it. While Skip was certain a cure was just around the corner, the wiser and more practical Dr. Cutter enumerated that a single magic bullet was unlikely and that progress on certain cancers like Skip's could be slow.

On this particular trip to 5 South, it was an unusually beautiful spring day and it just so happened to be the week of the Masters Golf Tournament. Skip had attended the Masters the year before with his friend Joe Roseburg. How a year could change one's life, Skip thought. Joe had hepatitis when he and Skip attended American University. Joe was a budding attorney at the Washington College of Law at American University, while Skip was working on his MBA at the Kogod School of Business. The hepatitis required Joe to have several blood transfusions. This was in the early '80s, prior to the advent of blood being screened for new infectious diseases. Unfortunately, one of the transfusions had injected Joe with HIV. His fight for survival lasted many years, but he finally succumbed that same year Skip was diagnosed. The ride to the hospital was bittersweet that particular day. Unbeknownst to Skip, he, too, would need blood transfusions to survive.

✝

On this trip to 5 South, Skip was given, among several other drugs, the drug Adriamycin, referred to as the "red devil" in chemo circles. It was by far the worst of the lot and difficult to face. In fact, in later treatments, Skip asked the nurses to put a pillow case over the red bag of poison so he didn't have to look at it flow. Just the sight of the chemical sent Skip reeling and pressing the nurse's button for extra nausea medicine. Visits in the hospital from friends and family were few and far between. Ashley was busy at home, and his friends and colleagues seemed to have their own lives going full tilt. Anyway, it didn't really matter; Skip was usually so sick or so out of it that he wouldn't have enjoyed the company anyway. Skip rarely left his room, but often he would feel the need to stretch out his legs or find a nurse who wasn't responding to his beeper. Did those beepers really work? Anyone who has been to a hospital wonders whether those beepers to the nurses' station are really connected. Even though the economy was tight, it was a little unnerving to have the same nurse taking your blood as well as emptying the trash cans.

During his infrequent hallway walks, Skip would occasionally run into another patient either out in the hall or walking to the nurses' station. On one such occasion, Skip was walking to the nurses' station to see if he could get an Ensure to drink, when he saw a nurse with a Budweiser beer can in her hand. He wasn't sure if it was time for "happy hour" on the floor or what. Not that Skip had the stomach for a beer at the moment, but it piqued his interest to see who was drinking on the floor. Wasn't this a chemo ward, thought Skip, and not the Copacabana? If an Advil ran $5.50 apiece, that Bud must be costing at least $100! Skip wondered if it was covered by insurance. It turns out that the beer was being delivered to a patient, a crusty old sort with a generous smile who welcomed Skip into the room. The gentleman in the room was also a patient of Dr. Barker. Names were exchanged but quickly forgotten by Skip, who never did have a memory for names. Faces were a different story. The old man told Skip that Dr. Barker had written him a prescription for two Budweisers a day. The nice old man offered one of his two to Skip, who politely declined. The thought of drinking alcohol was about as appealing as chewing lead chips. Skip and the old man became friends and met frequently in the elder's room. It was spring and the old man was a big Red Sox fan, and Skip would often walk with chemo pole in hand down to his room to catch a game and watch the Budweiser being consumed. The old man had some type of blood cancer and appeared to be a semipermanent member of 5 South. Skip would regularly look in on him on his biweekly visits.

Skip had returned to the hospital for another week of treatment and decided to force himself out of bed and take a walk to see what the old man was up to. There was a game on that night and Skip was feeling down and thought he might use some company. On approaching the old man's room, it was instantly apparent that something had changed. The bed was made and the television was off, with no sign of the old man. Skip thought that perhaps they moved him to another room or that he was undergoing some type of MRI or other test on another floor. Skip waddled to the nurses' station to inquire about the old man. The nurse told Skip that he wouldn't be coming back; he had died in his sleep two nights ago. He had finally succumbed to the disease. To be a patient on 5 South or any cancer floor brought an innate comradery among its patients. They all had something in common, though it was something they did not want. Hence, a fraternity of sorts. Even though he knew the old man for only a few months, they had quickly bonded and had become friends and cohorts against the disease. It was difficult to control his emotions in such an environment. The majority of the time sadness was the devil's tool. Other than an occasional visit with a fellow patient or pleasant conversation with one of the nurses, there was no happiness on 5 South, only agony. But it made the short time Skip spent with the old man all the more special. They were brief moments of pleasure mingled with a deluge of grief. Skip, his eyes welling with tears, went back to his room. A new wave of despair was rising. It would be a long night.

✝

Skip was roughly three months into the chemo regimen, and its effects were beginning to take a toll, not only on him but on the family as well. When Skip returned home from one of his biweekly hospital visits, he contributed little around the house. It put a strain on Ashley, who was taking care of the kids, Skip, and working full-time an hour from home. Long days and even longer nights were beginning to show in her personality. She became colder and more distant as time elapsed. At this point, the help from neighbors and the church had really subsided. The small church group that was coming over on a somewhat regular basis had stopped visiting, and Skip couldn't blame them. Skip wanted no part of company or conversation, which probably aided in the deteriorating relationships. Besides, he was either sick or in bed when folks from the church came over. As the prepared meals disappeared and the rides to the hospital became less frequent, Ashley was laden with even more.

Ashley would occasionally have a few friends over to try to maintain some sort of social life. Sometimes Skip would take part, but most of the time he was too nauseous or tired to participate. On one particular late afternoon, Ashley had the Gorhams and a couple of friends over from the Bay Club neighborhood. Caroline was in kindergarten at the time, and Foster had just begun to move around on his own. It was a beautiful late spring day. The views from the deck of the Sibleys' house were enviable and never grew tiresome. The tides played a large role in the landscape of the back of the house. Every hour of every day, the view was different based upon the position of the tides. It went from one striking extreme to another. When the tide was ebb, the marsh flowed with colorful grasses of varying shades of green. Conch creek was the closest body of water, winding its way to the Intracoastal Waterway in the far distance. It was breathtaking. We had often watched the herons arrive on queue as their internal biorhythms brought them into the marshland to feed upon the fiddler crabs and other delights as the tide had waned. The other end of the tidal spectrum occurred when the tide was high and water would overflow from the creek and the waterway to flood the marsh and bring new life into the ecosystem. Depending upon the moon and its lunar cycles, there could be vast amounts of water backing up into the Bay Club marsh-front homes. With the flood tide came the sea life. Smaller mud minnows, shrimp, and whatever bait fish abounded during a particular season all rolled into the marsh like clockwork. The smaller marine life brought in red drum, mullet, trout, and the occasional dolphin, depending on how much water flooded the marshscape. Regardless of the time of day, the vistas from behind the home were always in motion with ever-changing beauty and life. Skip was an avid fisherman and would take Caroline with him whenever he could. When the tide was high, the red drum came into the shallow flats looking for fiddler crabs and other bait fish. One could see them do what is called "tailing," as one assumes they are digging the shallow bottom for food, and one can see only their tail sticking out of the water. This is also known as sight fishing because you only cast for the fish you can see. Every so often when the tide was right, before his illness, Skip would grab his rod and Caroline and walk into the marsh grass looking for tailing red fish. Although they hooked one now and then, it was more about the sheer enjoyment of being on the water with his daughter, relishing the time they spent together.

On this particular late afternoon, the Gorhams and the other guests were all enjoying the vistas from the back deck, which sprawled from one end of the house to the other. The architect who built the house said, tongue-in-cheek, the deck space was large enough to land a helicopter. The house was two and a half stories, with another smaller deck on the top floor, which offered views that could take one's breath away. It was time for supper, so everyone went inside except for Foster and Skip. The smell of food did not agree with Skip, so he thought he would stay outside, watching the baby and the dog play. The weather was warm this particular afternoon, and Foster was wearing, for some reason, just a shirt with no diaper. As luck would have it, Foster did his business on the deck. Skip went inside quickly to see if anyone was interested in helping pick up Foster's "number two." Skip and Ashley came back out on the deck with paper towels and a bucket of water to clean the mess. Skip showed Ashley the spot, but the poop was gone. Skip was certain it was in that general area of the deck, but they couldn't find anything. Ashley looked at Foster, who was unfazed by it all, and then she looked at Trovo. Trovo was still licking his lips, enjoying the last morsels of Foster's deposit on deck. Man's best friend.

✝

The big bang theory or creationism? How was the universe formed? Immense questions with no verifiable answers. Scientists go in one direction and those of faith go in another. Skip would like to think that the beauty that was abundant around him could be sketched only by the hand of God. No mere circumstance created the tides that created the beauty of the marsh and ocean, he would say. While there is urban blight and immeasurable ghetto in the world now, nothing but beauty and awe existed in the beginning. Skip's world was changing, and so was his faith in God. He had nothing to lose but to believe.

Chapter 8

THE BANK IS OPEN

✝

Skip and Ashley had two beautiful, healthy children already. The doctors told Skip prior to the chemotherapy that if he and Ashley were interested in continuing to grow the family, there would be a problem. Skip's chemotherapy drug protocol would render him sterile and unable to procreate in the future. At this time, Ashley was not sure whether or not they should have more children. Of course they had talked about another child, but they had never pursued the idea seriously. Before the chemo regimen began, they both spoke with Dr. Barker who advised them of the one option available: a sperm bank. It really was no big deal, but the matter came down to cost. Between the visits and the storage, we were talking about a thousand dollars a year on average. The sperm was to be stored in a sperm bank in Augusta, Georgia. Maybe if they had a boy from there, he would be the next Tiger Woods.

The Sibleys decided to go with saving the sperm, just in case. The whole sperm bank experience was a little creepy for Skip. The Center for Reproductive Health was located in Charleston and appeared to be very professional. Inside Skip was greeted by a lovely receptionist who told him to take a seat and someone would be with him shortly. Within minutes, an even lovelier young woman greeted Skip and showed him to the doctor's office. Skip actually never saw a doctor on this visit but performed his duty and the future Sibley was sent off to be put on ice in a sperm bank in Augusta.

✝

Skip wasn't sure about much these days. He had lost all his hair from the chemo. His mother-in-law gave him his final trim before it was all gone. Skip looked like an Olympic swimmer, at least hair wise. In fact, he was totally hairless from head to toe. Skip knew that this was coming, but until the moment it arrived, he had held on to some hope that it wouldn't happen to him. And he was anything but an Olympian. He was growing more ill, and Ashley was growing more distant. She was spending more and more time at the office and less time at home. She would race to pick up Caroline at the after-school program and then hustle over to the nursery to get Foster before they closed. Skip was semi-oblivious to all this. Time had little meaning each day. He had his own marathon, and each day completed was a victory of sorts.

As usual, the first thing Caroline did upon returning home was run into the room and see Daddy. She was accustomed to his condition and loved him unconditionally all the same. They'd talk about her big day in kindergarten and anything else that was on her mind. If there was joy amidst the sorrow, this was part of it. God opened the skies and let their souls connect for these brief, precious moments, but it would bind them together as father and daughter forever. Caroline grew and matured at probably a much faster rate because of Skip's illness. She was alone more than usual and had chores that other children her age were unaware of. She was just a baby, but she would help with baby Foster. She fed him, read to him, and was a surrogate mother when Ashley was gone or busy. Caroline continued to grow more beautiful each day, with her long-flowing blond hair and beautiful brown eyes. Skip was amazed at the glory that God had created.

But the illness was taking its toll on Skip. He tried to maintain as ordinary a life as possible for the children, especially Caroline. Occasionally she would bring home math or reading that she wanted her dad to help with, but Skip had trouble doing basic math and was often unable to count to ten. Dr. Barker called it "chemo daze," whereby certain parts of the brain are affected by the drugs. How ironic. Skip had an MBA in finance and was now struggling with kindergarten math.

†

They called her Ms. Janie. One day Skip woke up and thought he was back in the antebellum South. He smelled warm, sweet potato pies and collard greens coming from the kitchen. The heavens opened up and dropped Ms. Janie on the doorstep when they needed help the most. Ms. Janie, you see, was the quintessential Southern Mammy to the Sibleys now. Skip never really questioned her arrival; he just assumed that she was sent from God, or she was sent by one of the neighbors down the street. Ms. Janie always had a calmness about her and put those around her at ease. She was filled with the Holy Spirit and loved to talk about Jesus, her family, or what Skip should be doing to get better. Although the topic never came up, Skip assumed that Ms. Janie was uneducated, at least in a formal manner. Skip with his MBA and Ms. Janie with her basic knowledge seemed odd companions.

Ms. Janie was black with long, dark black hair that she usually wore tied back. She was tall, about the size of Skip in stature, and was on the thin side. Skip couldn't imagine how she could gain any weight at all at the pace she kept up each day. She not only took care of Skip's family, but helped with one of the families down the road, and she also had a sister who lived with her who needed a lot of her attention. Ms. Janie would care for and converse with Skip as she went about her daily chores. Ms. Janie had the kind of wisdom that couldn't be learned from a textbook. She possessed a practical knowledge that was passed down to her through the generations. As with most Charlestonian black folks, her ancestors were slaves from Africa and ended up in the slave markets of the South Carolina Lowcountry. Skip, who had assumed she was literate because she spoke of Bible verses on a regular basis, was positioned well theologically between West Cooper Church and the Holy Spirit of Ms. Janie.

✝

The growth in nondenominational churches was prolific. The combination of a personalized homily and contemporary worship music was God's formula to let these types of churches develop and thrive. West Cooper was one such church. From humble beginnings in a local movie theatre to mega church in about a decade was proof that the formula worked. The church had bought land and built as it needed to sustain the growth in parishioners. From three hundred souls to over three thousand and multiple campuses, the blueprint for increasing the flock was a success at West Cooper. The head pastor, Greg Wood, had a personality in the pulpit that was unmatched. His sense of humor and modern-day message seemed to tug at churchgoers week after week. It was by the grace of God that he was given this ability, as he possessed a more introverted personality off the stage. Conversation was often difficult and shyness abounded, which made one feel almost uncomfortable in his presence. His place in leadership at the church was unquestioned. He was a star of the Lord and single-handedly helped the seekers find their way. If the words of the pastor were not enough, the praise and worship music that began and ended each service was the icing on the cake. Historic hymns gave way to contemporary Christian music that sounded as if one were at a rock concert. Although the music was loud and modern, the lyrics conveyed messages that were truly biblical, and it had a great deal to do with the growth of the church. The congregation couldn't get enough of this communion, so the church added special Wednesday services that were almost exclusively praise and worship music, services that were probably filled with more of the inner core of the church congregation. On Sunday one might see a few hands waving in the air to the music. But on Wednesday, the crowd stood the entire time with hands and arms raised to the sky praising the Lord. Guitars ablaze and melodic voices mesmerized the crowd. The service, usually the same each Wednesday, began with a brief prayer by the pastor, and then the band played several up-tempo songs before slowing it down to music in a softer tone. At this point, the pastor walked on stage and delivered a brief message to the audience, followed by communion. Skip remembered that the communion had freshly baked bread that was used to represent the body of Christ. He often wondered, especially during the cold and flu season, how people could drink from the same cup of the blood of Christ. He preferred to dip his bread in the cup to fulfill his rite of communion. Skip presumed that God would not let those who drank from the cup be afflicted with any ailment as a result of such drinking.

Over time, Skip took to West Cooper Church. It wasn't easy at first. Growing up in the Catholic Church was a world away from West Cooper, and it left many scars on Skip's religious memory. The legalism and the nuns haunted Skip for years. Many Catholics growing up and going to parochial school in the '60s and '70s shared these same emotions. Skip attended Our Lady of Lourdes Catholic School and was subjected to treatment that provided a plethora of sleepless nights in anticipation of going to school the following day. In those days, all classes were taught by nuns. One would only expect that someone who had dedicated her life to the worship of God and his love would share that same love with the students. This couldn't be further from the truth. Before the cancer and the chemotherapy introduced Skip to hell on Earth, he had a mild debriefing in such hellish experiences at Lourdes. No, the love of the Lord was not reciprocated to the minions who attended the school. Rather than being comforted by God's grace, they were condemned with sin and guilt that children of this age couldn't possibly understand.

Skip was small for his size and, at any age, this can be particularly painful, but as a young boy the teasing hurt more than a bee sting. At lunchtime, Skip would go through the line and get his hot lunch and sit at a table. Well, actually he sat on his knees so he could reach the tabletop in order to eat his food. "No, no, no," the nuns scolded. "We will have none of this." Skip was routinely hit with a ruler whenever he was caught sitting on his knees at the lunch table. The knees, said the nuns, were only for genuflecting in chapel for the Lord. Mimi and Maria then began making Skip a lunch to bring to school each day. At first it was several times a week, and then it turned into almost a daily occurrence where Skip was bringing his lunchbox home with his lunch untouched. Maria and Mimi would ask him why he hadn't touched his lunch, and Skip would respond that he wasn't hungry at that particular time of the day. Maria and Mimi decided to look into the situation a little further.

✝

Ms. Janie seemed to come and go like the wind. She worked irregular hours and was there some days but not others. Her conversations were lively, and Skip enjoyed the time spent with her. Her gabbing never precluded her from working. She was always dusting, cleaning, or performing some sort of household chore while keeping the conversation going. Skip was going through a phase where he tried to eat right and approach his disease with the aid of nutritional supplements and other alternative treatments. He brewed his essiac tea and drank it on a regular basis. Ms. Janie said that when she was young, she used to take bark off a certain type of tree and make it into a tea that would help particular ailments. She was an encyclopedia of alternative care that Skip tapped into on a regular basis. In the times before chemotherapy and radiation, people used elements of nature to cure disease. Skip thought that this art had long been lost but was reevaluating his stance after many a discussion with Ms. Janie.

When one's odds of survival are not good, one's natural tendency is to seek help from as many directions as possible. At least, that was Skip's game plan. Nothing was off the table or too extreme if it held the possibility to cure his cancer. Skip began experimenting modestly with supplements, herbs, and various tinctures that were purported to have some healing benefits. The problem was, if it was a problem at all, was that none of these so-called alternative treatments were approved by many, if any, doctors, nor the Food and Drug Administration. David Gorham would come over surprised at all the stuff Skip was taking and doing. (David came from the "laughter is better for healing" school of thought.) A man of means, David had said that he would send over clowns, penguins, midgets, or anything that would make Skip laugh. "Doesn't laughter add a decade or so to your life?" asked Gorham. The two shared countless episodes of laughter on the topic.

✝

Mimi took a part-time job at Lourdes as one of the lunch ladies to see if they could get to the bottom of the problem with Skip and his inability to eat lunch on a daily basis. None of this was ever mentioned to Skip, of course. He was not only small, but he was also shy. He must have gone through the lunch line for at least a week before he discovered that Mimi was behind the counter serving the kids. Those were the days when smoking was in vogue, Skip thought, as he remembered several of the lunch ladies with cigarettes in hand or mouth while doling out the food. Skip asked Maria if that was really Mimi working in the cafeteria at school. Maria told Skip that Mimi was such a good cook that they needed her help at Lourdes for a while. Skip never thought twice about it.

Recess at Lourdes had all the amenities of a federal prison: one parking lot and one ball. If this wasn't child cruelty, God only knows what was. Recess was his time to be tormented by the other boys for being short and sitting on his knees through lunch. Those boys weren't to blame; they were just mimicking what they saw in the classroom.

After serving lunch each day, Mimi would sneak a peak into the cafeteria and look for Skip to see if she could make heads or tails of this lunch dilemma. As if on queue, one of the nuns, Sister Sympathetic, as she was dubbed by the student body, rolled over to Skip and gave him a good whack on the back of his legs while he was sitting on his knees trying to eat his Friday fish and rice meal. Mimi had seen enough. She reported her findings to Maria who was shocked. The following day, Maria met with the principal to discuss the situation. After a short but poignant conversation, this was to be Skip's last day at Lourdes. Skip began a new elementary school life just down the road at a public school called Lynbrook, where he seemed to thrive.

✝

Skip's taste for the alternative in cancer treatments was reaching new heights. His sister-in-law, Toni, and her mother Sandy were well-versed in alternative healing. Sandy at one point even owned her own health food store. When they came to visit Skip, not only did they bring books and vitamins, they also brought a wealth of information that would have taken years to assemble, even with the Internet. Sandy was especially skilled at the art of reflexology, which she performed on Skip several times. Reflexology is a therapeutic foot message that uses key pressure points that correspond to various parts of the body. It is a relaxing and wonderful experience. If chemotherapy was on one end of the treatment scale, then reflexology would be close to the other end.

When he had the energy, Skip pored over books that Toni and Sandy brought. He also used Internet search engines to garner any information that might be helpful. The world of naturopathy or holistic healing had been around forever, but it was now making its way into the mainstream and into Skip's vernacular. The world of vitamins, supplements, and herbal remedies were all lumped together by Skip in his efforts to find data on any that might help with his cancer. As one can imagine, there was no magic bullet or particular vitamin that targeted Skip's rare form of bone cancer, but there were nutritional supplements that helped the immune system in general and were purported to have positive effects at fighting cancer cells. Skip's role and mind-set had to be as positive as possible in his search for a cure.

Ashley, on the other hand, had a more pragmatic approach. Data on Ewing's sarcoma was sparse, due to its rare nature. But the limited amount that existed was worth its weight in gold. Ashley found data from several major cancer institutions and publications. Although the information did not have large sample sets, the data nonetheless was important. Ashley discerned from the literature that the two main indicators of survival for a tumor of this type were its size and location in the body. Obviously, the larger the tumor, the harder it would be to treat. These tumors range in size from small micro bursts to tumors the size of grapefruits. Skip's tumor was roughly the size of a walnut in the bone in his right arm. Not terrible, but not great either. It was within the range that radiation and chemotherapy had a chance of working. The location of the tumor was also very significant. Organs generally offer a much worse prognosis than tumors found in soft tissue or bone. Skip's walnut-size tumor was located in the upper or proximal portion of the humerus bone in his right arm. Not the worst location, but not the greatest either. Additional factors, such as age and general health, weighed into the equation, but to a lesser extent.

A combination of the size and location categorized Skip as a stage II Ewing's sarcoma case, with the odds of survival less than 50 percent. Moreover, collateral damage to the right arm was almost guaranteed. But the longer he survived the cancer, the better his overall chances of going into remission. Skip didn't want to hear any of this. The prognosis based on Ashley's research was not optimal. In any case, Skip needed to do more than what the doctors were doing. He had to take the battle into his hands, or so he thought.

✝

The sermon hit Skip right in the heart, as it usually did, on this particular Sunday, something about Paul and suffering and bringing one closer to God. Skip shouldn't have been caught off guard when Pastor Greg asked the assembly if anyone had ever gone through a period of suffering. Just about every hand shot up in response, as they did to most of the rhetorical questions solicited from the pulpit. Skip wondered how Pastor Greg knew what he was feeling and that seemingly each week the homily would involve Skip's life in some fashion. West Cooper Church was large, but the pastoral staff was fairly accessible to the congregation. Skip had all the questions of those who endure difficult times. What will happen next? How will he take care of the family? How did he become afflicted with cancer? It didn't seem fair! Finances, health, relationships—the list went on and on. Surely a benevolent God would intervene and end the suffering. Skip was still a neophyte in regard to his walk with the Lord and had many more questions than answers. He just wanted to see his family grow. He wanted to see his daughter graduate and get married. He barely knew baby Foster, whose new life would help Skip garner strength and hope for the future.

Foster Sibley was baptized at West Cooper Church on a warm summer evening. It was the first significant event since Skip became ill, so he was counting his blessings that he was able to attend the baptism. Ashley was videotaping the ceremony for posterity. Skip was not generally good with crowds, but it appeared that every member of the church was having their child baptized this particular evening. Skip, Caroline, and Foster were on the stage with the others while Ashley videotaped from below. Caroline giggled at Foster when Pastor Greg referred to him as a girl instead of a boy. With a name like Foster and being like father, without hair, it was an honest mistake. Skip remembers looking at himself on the video. He had lost so much weight and so much hair, he hardly recognized himself. "Is that really me up there?" remarked Skip to himself while watching the video. He looked and felt like a cancer patient—a blue blazer hanging from a skeleton with a sling on its right arm, bald and spectacled. "What happened to the man I use to be?" But life continued. He still had to get up each morning and put on his shoes and do whatever needed to be done.

Skip's recent physical demise had its effects on him psychologically as well. He became self-conscious and even more introverted, bordering on agoraphobic. Traumatic events in Skip's life led to panic attacks ultimately manifesting into derealization. Was God allowing the devil to pull Skip's strings like a marionette? Skip was too close to the chaos and unable to see anything other than the present realm. The trauma of the last several months weighed heavily on Skip. It was difficult for him to go about any kind of routine without lapsing into dissociation about life, or death. Rest. Need sleep.

†

"Your tongue looks terrible," remarked the doctor of alternative medicine, who was about to perform acupuncture on Skip. Apparently, much could be told from the way a tongue looks and, according to the doctor, Skip was not looking good. He suffered extreme nausea from months of chemotherapy and radiation and heard that acupuncture might help his condition. The doctor was an actual medical doctor and not a naturopathic healer. He practiced at the Medical University of the South, and he performed a routine physical on patients prior to launching into the pins and needles. Skip was obviously in bad condition, with his ghostly appearance, bald head, and arm in a sling. The doctor surmised he was suffering from some sort of cancer. Skip concurred and told the doctor the story. No matter how many times Skip told the story of taking Caroline to the fair and getting on the ride and breaking his arm, it was like telling it for the first time. The response elicited by the story, too, was almost always the same: a mixture of incredibility and sympathy.

The first time a pin or needle enters one's body in the form of acupuncture is a little intimidating. Unlike a shot, which tends to come right out, this needle is inserted and resides there for what seems an eternity. Skip assumed that like reflexology, there were specific points of interest on the body where the pins were placed to perform their healing magic. Although acupuncture had been around for centuries, it was difficult to find someone to perform this art—or is it a science?—in the Charleston area. An act of God placed this doctor at the local university hospital at this time. He was doing rounds at various clinics and was in Charleston for a short time. Skip couldn't begin to imagine how many pins would be placed in his body that day, but his guess was somewhere around fifty, maybe more. When he got home that evening, Ashley asked Skip how it went. He said the usual, that he was a human pin cushion, but he felt a little better having done the treatment. Skip would have an acupuncture appointment pursuant to every chemo visit from this point forward.

Due to the severity of the damage to the arm, no type of physical therapy was attempted. Instead, Skip sought out chiropractic treatment to enhance his immune system and overall health. This world of medicine, especially the alternative side, was so new to Skip. But his experiences to date made him a big believer in the alternative arena. The chiropractic treatments also seemed to help Skip's overall physical and mental health. The downside was that the chiropractor wanted to see Skip at least three times a week. This was difficult to do and became somewhat expensive as well. Skip agreed to come twice a week and hoped to cut back to once per week after a month or so. The doctor was good and gentle with the arm and body and put Skip through various exercises, bends, cracks, and stretches. Skip even brought Caroline and Foster to the chiropractor, for it was said that chiropractic treatments could help with ear infections, a common problem for many babies like Foster. Skip wasn't keen to give Foster antibiotics for those infections, so the chiropractor performed several manipulations on Foster that seemed to help. A combination of these manipulations, which included tugging on the ear and a small amount of pain reliever took care of this and future ear infections for Foster. Skip took Caroline once or twice just to get an overall assessment of her chiropractic health, since she was a very active child and prone to injury. She checked out fine and would occasionally return as needed.

Diet consumed Skip's life. Between chemotherapy visits, he had made some drastic changes to what he was eating. Skip had no diet before cancer. He ate whatever he wanted. He was relatively thin and athletic, so he assumed that the inside of his body must be the same. He was certainly no candidate for type II diabetes, but other degenerative diseases could lurk in even the healthiest-looking bodies. The diet was a difficult balancing act. Since there was such a dramatic weight loss, the doctors told Skip to eat whatever he could to keep weight on. On the other side, everything alternative suggested that what Skip had been eating on a regular basis was bad, and could actually cause the immune system to let down and become vulnerable to illness. He began modestly by cutting out the sugars, white flour, and other alternative no-no's that were said to weaken the immune system. The best alternative to cancer was not getting it in the first place. However, once it becomes part of you, you must symbiotically associate cancer into your life. Since there is no cure for cancer, building up one's own bodily defenses through a powerful immune system was about the best alternative to traditional treatment. Although Skip still fantasized about Krispy Kreme doughnuts and mashed potatoes, in which he was still indulging, he would eventually turn to a more vegetarian lifestyle, ultimately culminating into a macrobiotic way of life.

Chapter 9

APPARITIONS AND

LOCUTIONS

✝

She was the wife of a preacher and became friends with Skip during chemotherapy visits. While they did not share the same doctors, they shared the same grief, sorrows, and occasional joy. She was a light-toned, young black woman in her late twenties or early thirties with short black hair and was suffering from a very malignant form of breast cancer. The only upside was that it didn't seem to affect her hair. She and her husband were only married a few years and, like Skip, were just celebrating the arrival of a new baby to their family. God seemed to be working his way into Skip's life from all avenues as time went on. What were the odds of Skip's taking chemo in a room next to a young pastor's wife? Her husband was soft-spoken, with a mild demeanor that had a calming effect on Skip. He visited his wife every day, so Skip looked forward to the opportunity to talk with him. The pastor brought an aura of hope to a part of the hospital that was generally hopeless. He encouraged Skip to be strong and courageous, for the Lord your God, quoting Deuteronomy he would say, will never leave you nor forsake you. Skip took extreme comfort in his words and wisdom, which helped alleviate the worry and anxiety.

Skip's visits with the pastor were brief, so Skip spent much of his time on good days speaking with the pastor's wife. While Skip held on to considerable doubt and worry about his healing, she was never concerned about death or dying and would always quote a verse of scripture that gave her strength and encouragement. God was going to heal her, she would say every time she and Skip spoke. They would always pray together, for one another. Both were young with growing families and had so much to live for. Surely God could see this and make their lives better, in order to enjoy the gifts, including childbirth, that they were given.

Breast cancer comes in many shapes and sizes, ranging on the scale of relatively benign to that of advanced malignancy. The pastor's wife had a very aggressive stage IV type of breast cancer that was tough to fight. Pursuant to a double mastectomy, she was on the most advanced chemotherapy protocol in an attempt to capture and kill any remaining cancerous cells. Her appearance began to diminish, with her countenance deteriorating each time they met. Skip could tell that she was growing weaker, and taking a turn for the worst. In the meantime, they kept praying for a cure.

✝

Prayer sessions for most were designed as a way to communicate with a deity. In the Christian faith, prayer can be a way to interact with God on a personal basis. Skip thought of his first locution during a prayer time while genuflecting to the Lord in response to his first hearing of the bad news of the Ewing's sarcoma diagnosis. This private revelation put a positive set of thoughts in Skip's mind as his prayers were being said. There was no doubt that these thoughts were from an outside source, and Skip fully believed that God was listening and responding through these locutions. One must be very careful when thoughts or ideas are placed in him or her from an external source. This is a trick of the devil as well. In general, if the locution is spiritual in the sense that it derives peace, hope, or some other positive factor, it can generally be thought of as answer to prayer. In Skip's case, his prayer was that he would give up control of his life and rely totally on the grace of God to get him through each event of each day. A task much easier prayed than done. At the time of the locution, however, Skip was certain that his prayers were being heard and answered from God in a positive way. Unbeknownst to Skip, this would be a short-term bottoming point in his life. The ladder had many rungs, and Skip was currently near the bottom. But he had the promise of God that, shortly, he'd climb higher.

✝

The pastor's wife paid a visit to Skip one evening after dinner at the hospital. Neither of them could really tolerate the food that was being served. It wasn't that the food was so terrible; they simply had little to no appetite due to the nausea caused by the chemo treatments. The meal selection had to include just the right item to invoke hunger. There was a slim chance that what one felt like eating would be served during that meal. Skip, being such a frequent guest, made good friends with the nursing staff. At times, they would actually call in the food nutritionist, and she would get Skip something to eat from outside the hospital to make him feel better. Skip was brought everything from Subway sandwiches to cheeseburgers from McDonald's. The pastor's wife would often visit Skip during dinner hours but would rarely partake in eating herself. She had lost so much weight and looked so fatigued most of the time that Skip was really beginning to worry about her. His recurring thought? Most patients never leave 5 South.

✝

He wasn't the hospital chaplain whom Skip knew very well. Rather, he was a minister of a church in Charleston who was making his rounds at the hospital, visiting patients. He stuck his head into Skip's room, and the two made eye contact, which was enough of an invite for the minister to enter the room and make Skip's acquaintance. They bantered small talk back and forth for a while before the minister got down to business. Speaking in tongues was the gift of this particular servant of God, and the minister imparted such teachings to Skip. Try as he might, Skip could not make heads or tails out of the whole situation of tongues, let alone the locutions that the minister said would and could be received during such times. As Skip was winding down his lesson in "Tongues 101," the minister's wife and another gentleman entered the hospital room and began speaking in tongues themselves. Skip thought the whole incident bizarre, but thanked them for coming. Skip made several vain attempts throughout the remainder of the day to summon the tongues himself but, alas, nothing.

✝

It was the end of what would normally be a business day, and Ashley and the kids visited Skip at the hospital this particular evening. Skip's week-long stint was just beginning, so he needed all the love and encouragement that could be mustered for him. Ashley brought the day's paper and a few magazines that might interest Skip during his down time. Foster was getting bigger every day, and Caroline would always make Daddy a card or some such trinket and bring it with her to the hospital to make Skip feel better. She looked adorable as she was still in her little school uniform during visits. Foster crawled around the floor of the room, but even though it was a hospital, something told Ashley the floors were not as clean as they were at home. Ashley would usually try to get Skip something to eat that he was craving on her way to the hospital. This particular night it was a barbeque plate from Momma Blacks, a local Charleston BBQ joint. It hit the spot. Skip left the hospital food tray of fish and rice untouched; it was taken back to the cafeteria by an elderly black woman. She asked Skip if he wasn't hungry, and he told her that dinner was brought in from the outside world tonight. She laughed and gave him a big smile and went on with the rest of her rounds.

Skip never felt much like reading, although he was an avid reader. While doing the chemo, between the nausea and fatigue, he had little desire to read. On this evening, he felt compelled for some reason to pick up the newspaper and thumb through it. When he got to the State and Local section, he froze and dropped the paper. Stunned, he picked up the paper and began again to read the headline about a pastor's wife who had just died of breast cancer. There was no mistaking the picture of the grieving preacher. It was his friend. The article went on to chronicle his ministry and her cancer and the family left behind. Skip read the article several times and then took a walk down the hall where her room used to be. He stood there in silent prayer remembering the pastor's wife. She was such a believer in Jesus and knew that she would be healed. Skip realized just then that when she spoke of being healed, this was metaphoric for being saved for eternity. Skip was still too young in his walk to understand completely. All he knew was that she was a preacher's wife with a direct pipeline to God. If God took her, what chance did Skip really have? Confusion reigned and emotions surfaced. Skip fell to the ground and had to be carried back to his bed by the nursing staff. He was mildly sedated and dozed in and out of a restless sleep.

†

The chemo treatments were in full swing with Skip about halfway through the process. On his off-hospital weeks, he'd attend church if he had the energy. One particular Sunday, he and the family sat up high in the upper deck. Skip wore a mask and wasn't really supposed to be around crowds of people, where he might contract some sort of virus or bug. With a depleted immune system and low white blood cell count, Skip had little ammunition to fight off infection of any kind. Like drinking from the chalice of wine, Skip did not believe that God would inflict harm on him while he attended a church service. Time was given during the service to a young woman who was running an orphanage in Romania. Complete with a slide show, details were divulged of how these poor children lived.

Tied to their beds, malnourished, and neglected, these children needed someone or some organization to step in and help them. Marcia King was on a one-woman campaign to make this happen. She was at West Cooper Church this particular weekend to get the word out about her project and solicit any kind or remuneration she could from the usually sympathetic congregation. Marcia had begun a project called Children Under the Son, which was set up as an orphanage; but it also was used as a ministerial outreach to the Romanian community. In addition, it served as a medical arm to help the orphans get hospital care if they were in need of some type of surgical procedure. After the presentation and at the conclusion of the sermon, Skip walked by the table where Marcia was set up to grab a brochure and make a donation. Marcia couldn't help but notice Skip's condition, and a conversation had begun. One thing led to another, and they exchanged phone numbers. Skip had ventured into the realm of mission work for the first time. The thought of helping others, especially children in despair, gave Skip some hope. Although he had yet to realize it, by helping others, he was also beginning to heal himself.

✝

Skip was back from a grueling visit to 5 South and lay in bed one early evening as the rest of the family was having supper. Skip felt like watching a little television, so he turned on the set. Skip was not a big TV watcher, as it usually just made noise that would end up making him more nauseous. This particular night something compelled him to turn on the TV and flip around to see what was on. While channel surfing, he stopped on a Christian broadcasting station. Inside of the set, staring right into Skip's eyes, was this man with a white suit and what looked like a gray toupee. He was ending his show, a show that Skip had never seen before, with prayer. There were no sheets of paper nor written prayer requests in front of him. It was as if God were telling him what to say to the audience. He went through a litany of prayer and finally opened his eyes and raised his head and looked directly into the camera at Skip, and said, "Lord, a young man will be healed of bone cancer." Benny Hinn had just spoken a healing prayer directly to Skip. Benny Hinn is best known for performing healing miracles through his evangelical ministry of some thirty-six years. Again, unbeknownst to Skip, this minister was a best-selling author and television evangelist. He was infamous in his worldwide healing organization. Skip couldn't believe his ears and eyes. Did that really just happen, or was he in another chemo daze? There was no way of knowing for sure, but Skip was a believer. He called feverishly for the rest of the family to come. When Ashley came, he told her that he had just been healed by the television. Ashley raised her eyebrows. Skip meant the man on the television, Benny Hinn. Skip told the story as Caroline raced into the room.

"Ashley, Benny Hinn just declared by the Word of God that a man will be healed from bone cancer," said Skip. "Can you believe it?"

Ashley didn't know what to say. She had never heard of Benny Hinn. But Caroline was ecstatic about the news of her daddy being better. Skip was certain this minister was referring to him. What are the odds that he would turn the TV on, flip around the channels, and feel compelled to stop on a station and show that he had never seen before? Skip wanted to see it again and again, but to no avail. Surely it was the hand of God who directed him in the direction of Benny Hinn. Hope is eternal, and Skip needed a great deal of hope at that particular time. Benny Hinn had just given him something to cling onto. Skip didn't care what anyone else said or thought about the Benny Hinn Ministries; he was a believer and nothing would change his mind.

✝

Marcia King was a beautiful young woman with sinuous dark hair, who was petitioned by God to become a missionary in a remote land. The town of Oradea, Romania, was ground zero for her efforts to heal a town and a war-torn land that still existed in the shadows of socialism. In effect, the orphanage was a microcosm of Romania itself. The futile attempts at economic reform offered the average Romanian only a minimal existence. The orphanage fostered the results of the neglect. Children by the dozens were abandoned weekly in Oradea alone, for life under a Godless, communist utopia had failed them and left them with sundry economic and social issues, causing this catastrophe. The orphanage was the crux of the trilogy of support being offered by Marcia and her band of in-country national helpers. The government-run hospitals and children's facilities would be enough to bring the average American to his or her knees. All types of neglect existed here, from lack of food and proper clothing, to outright pain and torture inflicted upon the homeless young. God by no means created situations like these, but he did create people like Marcia to fill the gap between heaven and hell on Earth.

A primary school enveloped the second layer of care at Children Under the Son, a school that cared not only for children raised at the orphanage, but also for children in the community who had been rejected by the local state schools for their positions in society. God again showed Marcia a need, and she and her group were there to fill it.

The third spoke in the wheel at Children Under the Son was a healing ministry for children. Success stories ranged from burn victims to brain injuries. The healing mission is generally the only hope for a family or child who requires medical attention. Obviously, these families have no money to pay for this kind of medical care, so Marcia and her group solicit funds from around the world to get the job done. Romania is a unique and wonderful land caught in a time lapse, leaving it fragile and unable to really move much beyond the status of third world.

†

St. Paul's apparition on the road to Damascus was an enigmatic happening that changed the course of the world forever. It is a well-known story in the book of Acts of Saul the tax collector and persecutor of early Christianity having a vision of Jesus and losing his sight, only to regain it by the hands of Ananias of Damascus. It may be the most profound, life-changing experience ever documented resulting from an apparition of Christ. Visions have existed for centuries in Christian society, ranging from Marian apparitions, witnessing the mother of Jesus, to Constantine's vision of Christ's sign in AD 312.

Although she was becoming more reclusive, Ashley was also becoming more interested in the Word of God. Not only was she reading the Bible, but she was also reading a daily devotional. Skip and Ashley did not often discuss their religious beliefs together. Skip didn't even know that she was becoming so involved until she told him about an event the night before. Unlike Skip's wild excitement in regard to the Benny Hinn message, Ashley was more reserved in the sharing of her story.

✝

Mimi was in her early nineties and living in a nursing home after years of wonderful care from Maria and Mack. She had been declining steadily over the last several years, with bouts of memory loss and other issues related to growing old. Mimi lived a good and peaceful time on this earth and, beyond the expectations of many, had lived a number of years after Dominic's death. Mimi passed away peacefully in her sleep at the nursing home one cool spring night. God had decided it was time to take this good and faithful servant of the Lord home to rest for eternity.

It was anything but restful with the rest of the family. Mimi was loved by all. She had outlived her other nine siblings and friends, so Maria and Donnie's family were all that she had left. Ashley received the news from Maria but was afraid to tell Skip that Mimi had died. Skip was very close to Mimi and actually lived with her for several years while going to graduate school. Those were some of Skip's fondest memories. Mimi had been a great cook and Skip and his friends took advantage of it at every opportunity. Mimi retained her skills, but memory loss and fatigue had diminished her quality of life, and her ability to prepare meals. One particular afternoon when he was waiting to leave for an afternoon class at American University, Mimi was going to make him a quick sandwich before he left. The dining room was small but was occupied by a rather large mirror that could be seen from any seat at the dining room table. Mimi brought out the sandwich and chips for Skip, and as he lifted the sandwich to his mouth, he happened to glance up at the mirror, instantly dropping the sandwich to the plate. What Skip had seen was a piece of bread that was dark green from mold on the bottom slice of his ham and cheese. Skip never mentioned the incident to Mimi, as it would have broken her heart. Instead he told her he would eat the rest in the car. Skip quietly discarded the sandwich over the fence to the neighbor's German shepherd. Then, he made a conscious note to himself to always scan the plate before eating with Mimi.

The news hit Skip like a ton of bricks. He wasn't feeling well anyway, and he could barely comprehend what Ashley was saying. Skip was so wrapped up in his own issues that he hadn't spent that much time thinking about Mimi. The two hugged and cried over their loss. Mimi was the last of the old school generation, with roots in Europe and memories of good days long past.

†

Skip was still grieving over the loss of Mimi and was determined, though he knew better, to attend the funeral. This would require missing chemo, getting on a crowded and potentially germ-infested plane, and flying to Delaware. He knew deep down that he wouldn't be able to go.

Ashley sat on the couch in the kitchen as she did on most nights, reading her daily devotional during a peaceful time when the house was finally at rest. The apparition came as swiftly as it went away. A woman in white, very bright white, appeared before Ashley, hovering slightly above the ground. The woman was unmistakable and had a physical transparency about her that made her look ghost-like. Ashley was never afraid, but had an incredible sense of peace at the vision of Mimi's presence hovering over her. Ashley wasn't sure how long Mimi was there before she spoke to her. Mimi was magnificent with brilliant white features and pleasant countenance. When Mimi spoke, Ashley was stunned. It was almost like Mimi was illuminated in the air from a projector. Words were spoken not from her mouth, but rather from her presence. Mimi said to her, "God knows that you and Skip are struggling with my death, and that Skip is heartbroken about not being able to attend my funeral. Know that it is alright and peace be with you, for your God is a great and almighty God." And just like that, it was over. Similar to Skip and his encounter with

Benny Hinn, Ashley sat stunned, wondering if the event she just witnessed really happened. Skip was sleeping as Ashley crawled into bed beside him; she decided not to wake him, that he could hear the story in the morning. As one could imagine, Ashley didn't sleep at all that evening, replaying the vision of Mimi over and over in her head until she heard the alarm clock go off. She must have dozed off as it was time for work and another day. She was up and had the kids ready and out of the house before Skip awoke.

Later that evening, Ashley sat Skip down and told him of the vision of Mimi. These were very trying times for Skip. The chemo was wearing him to near death, and the loss of Mimi was another huge factor in his declining health. Skip was exuberant over the apparition and firmly believed that it was real. He needed to hear this. It came at a time when he was ready to give up on life, family, and all. The day-to-day struggle was just too much. He couldn't eat and lost so much weight. Those were endless days of post-chemo, of receiving blood transfusions at the hospital. Skip wanted to be with Mimi in a place where there was no more pain. He had grown weary of the earth and was searching now for the transcendent. However, this news from Ashley was quite unbelievable, and it gave Skip hope to carry on, at least for a little while longer.

✝

Skip became friends with Marcia and helped her with various stateside affairs. Marcia spent most of the year in Romania, so she needed help with basic things like banking, shipping supplies, and other activities that required one to be in the United States. A board of directors was put together, and Skip was elected chairman for Children Under the Son. The remainder of the group was made up of local parishioners from West Cooper. The main function of the board was to get Marcia the money and supplies needed from the United States to Romania, which was no easy task. Fundraising was always taking place, whether it was among board members or on one of Marcia's trips back to America. Once, they received donations from the church and community that filled one entire tanker container that would eventually get shipped to Romania. Like everything, it took time and money to organize, but after seeing the neglect of the poor children, it made it impossible not to push events forward.

Romania has changed little in the time that Skip has been involved with Children Under the Son. Orphans abound, and government hospitals are still subpar. Only a society fearless of a greater God could allow these injustices. How could someone allow a baby to lie in a bed for weeks on end, being tied to a crib, never being changed, and never knowing human touch? What kind of soulless individual could watch the malnourishment and tortuous treatment of children? Marcia would ask these questions of the women working in these facilities, and they would only shrug and say they were doing the best they could with what little they had. To an outsider it was incomprehensible how this could all go on. God bless Children Under the Son.

✝

The mystical door to the heavens opened again for the Sibleys. Skip was very sick from the chemo and could barely hold down any food. He weighed less than 140 pounds and was dropping weight rapidly. The doctors were not pleased with his condition, although there had been nothing but positives to take away from Skip's recent x-rays, MRIs, and other tests. It was the chemotherapy that was kicking his butt. At this point, there were no surprises in regard to the chemo protocol. Skip arrived at the hospital, checked in, and waited for the nurse to administer his concoction of poison. An IV bag was filled with medicine and hung by his bedside. Medicine was injected into his life port that was surgically implanted in his chest. That was the easy part. In the beginning, these visits were new to him, varying slighting in intensity and agony. But he knew what was coming next. It's like knowing that your hand is going to be slammed in the car door. You see it coming, but you can't stop it. Each drop from the IV brought on new levels of pain. His body was wearing down physically and mentally. Skip didn't know if he had the strength to continue with the treatments. His meals were nonexistent, and his diet consisted of drinking Ensure whenever the nurses would bring it to him. His days of visiting other patients were over. He had neither the strength nor the desire to enlist the company of anyone. Where are you, God? Why must I suffer so? Is this all part of a larger plan? These were the questions he asked himself regularly. Not so different from what Jesus was thinking on the cross in his final hours, asking the Father if there was another way. Was it all worth it? Peace without pain was all he wanted. Jesus walked this way two thousand years ago and took a seat at the right hand of the Father. Skip wanted to be in heaven with Jesus and be at peace. He knew that he had a family and earthly duties, but as his mind grew weary, even these things were pushed aside in an effort to find a painless environment. The only one that Skip knew of was heaven.

Again, it happened in an instant, but its effects would persist. Ashley was sitting on the couch in the kitchen area when the apparition took place. Just prior to the appearance, she was praying for Skip and the pain to ease, and reading her devotional. Ashley knew from a recent visit to Dr. Barker that Skip was not well, and his chances of making it through the chemo were not good. Peace. Peace filled the air of the quiet home that late evening. Ashley was trancelike in her countenance, with a complete feeling of relaxation encompassing her. Similar to the apparition of Mimi, it took place so quickly. But the white light that shone was a hundred times brighter this time. At first, Ashley was blinded by the brilliance of the light but, slowly her eyes adjusted and focused on the figure before her. The apparition at first was not clear; she couldn't make out who or what it was. Like Mimi, though, the light hovered above the kitchen floor, touching neither the ground nor the ceiling. Ashley's mind was racing. While she was at peace, she didn't know what was happening or what might be coming. Suddenly, the light began taking form; it was the shape of a man. Ashley now knew that this was something special—ordinary people being presented with miraculous situations. Who was she to be allowed to experience this? What seemed long gone and left to the Old Testament, encounters with the Holy One did not happen in this generation. Then He spoke. "Peace be with you, my child." Ashley's eyes fixated on the apparition as God spoke again. "Peace be with you, for it is not his time." Then silence. The aura of God lingered but remained silent. Ashley had no idea how much time had elapsed. And then, God spoke again, "Peace be with you, my child, for it is not his time to be with me." Tears of joy streamed down Ashley's face.

✝

Skip was in the hospital when the vision took place but, almost simultaneously, peace had also come over him. Again, Ashley had a sleepless night reflecting on the apparition. But on Saturday morning, she raced down to the hospital to tell Skip of the wonderful news. Skip was again elated and amazed and didn't know what to think. Ashley wanted to tell Skip more of the encounter, but it happened so suddenly and was so remarkable that she was lost in the moment. She also had a difficult time describing what she saw, although the words were unmistakable. The vision was brighter than light, with the figure of what looked to be a man coming and going in and out of sight. Afterward, the aura of peacefulness remained, and Ashley basked in it.

Skip told Ashley that he had an unusually peaceful presence come over him last night as well. So many questions with so few answers, but this is what Skip desired to keep his spirits alive and moving forward. Ashley was the bearer of blessings again, and they came at just the right moment—a visit and words from the Creator. How unimaginable and unbelievable. Skip was close to telling Dr. Barker that he couldn't handle the chemo any longer and wanted to end it, but this news had changed everything. He still didn't understand why God had him suffer so, but there must be an end. So, he had righted the boat and began sailing in a better direction. Skip and Ashley were just two, regular people raising kids and working until the tragedy entered their lives. Surely God didn't have the time to communicate with all those who were suffering and in pain in this world. Or did he?

Chapter 10
LYING IN DARKNESS

†

He had had enough; that was the consensus. There is a fine line between giving a patient too much chemotherapy to kill the cancer cells and causing havoc on other parts of the body. Dr. Barker had decided to call it quits. Skip was three days into his seven-day hospital stay when Dr. Barker shared the news. Skip's blood counts and other measures were way too low to keep up the chemo protocol. The Adriamycin alone was known to cause serious heart damage if given in extreme doses. All of this meant pulling the plug on the rest of the chemo treatments. Skip had another month or so to go before completing the predetermined cycle. Tears rolled down Skip's face when he heard the news from Dr. Barker. But was it enough? The St. Jude's protocol suggested a longer duration. Were all the cancer cells dead and gone? These and other issues began to worry Skip. It didn't matter, though. He was done. He had endured a little over a year of hell on earth, and now that it was over Skip put his faith in God, and Dr. Barker, that this was the right move.

Skip called Ashley at the office to tell her the good news, although he couldn't get a hold of her at that moment. He left a message to call him back, as he wanted to tell her the news in person. It was over. It was finally over. The chemo was done and would not be used again. Bullets number one and two were exhausted. Skip had maxed out on the amount of radiation that a person can endure in one lifetime. If there were a reoccurrence, radiation therapy would not be an option. The downside to more radiation was the increased risk of more cancer, believe it or not. Too much radiation, Dr. Barker explained, could lead to additional sarcomas in the future. No more radiation!

Bullet number two, the chemotherapy, was also exhausted. Too much poison medicine was not good for the body. Issues surrounding various organs, especially the heart, liver, and kidneys, were at risk of overdosing on the chemo. Skip had maxed out on phase two of his treatment against the disturbing Ewing's sarcoma.

He and Ashley discussed the prospects and decisions were made. Radiation—done. Chemotherapy—over. Ashley was hoping that the end of the chemo would lift Skip's spirits. He had been beaten down for so long that he was just a remnant of his former self. Once the chemo purged itself from his body, he might regain an appetite and put on some of the weight that he had lost during the treatments. Skip looked like a POW, with no hair and an emaciated body. He felt like a POW as well.

†

The journey to Duke Medical Center was much more welcoming, in a sense, than that of their previous visits. This time Skip and Ashley thought they would make a long day trip out of it because of the kids, and they didn't want to bother the Claytons again. A lifetime ago it seemed that Skip was at Duke listening to the doctors explain his upcoming chemotherapy. At that time, Skip did not know what they meant by aggressive chemotherapy. But now he was done and a veteran of such treatment. After the chemotherapy and radiation treatment, the doctors at Duke ordered a battery of tests, among them a PET scan to see if any additional cancer was present. The PET scan and all the other tests and x-rays came back negative, much to the relief of Skip and Ashley. Now, phase three was about to begin.

The usual series of treatment for Ewing's sarcoma was radiation, chemotherapy, and surgery. Phase three was surgery. This was at the crux of his conversation with Dr. Laurie at Duke. He was the chief orthopedic oncologist on staff and examined Skip without Ashley being present. It was his opinion that the arm had to go. Well, at least the humerus bone and perhaps a portion of the scapula. Skip felt nauseated as the conversation continued. Hadn't he already been through enough? Weren't the scans and tests all negative? Why should he have to endure another procedure?

Dr. Laurie had insinuated that the bone in Skip's arm had become too compromised, so it would be better to replace it now before it broke again. Duke was a major cancer center and at the forefront of clinical care in cancer throughout the country. As such, Dr. Laurie's statement had floored Skip. The latest and greatest technology at Duke was replacing Skip's current arm with a cadaver arm and bone! Even Dr. Laurie painted a tainted picture of the surgery. The risk of infection and Skip's body rejecting the implant were very high. The cadaver arm, at best, would give Skip minimal use of his right arm. However bad it sounded, it surely beat the alternative—amputation. Just ten years ago, amputation was the method of choice to dispose of the cancerous bone in the arm. How wonderful. Science had progressed so much in a decade that the only solution was amputation. Once again, Skip was hit with a one-two punch by the medical profession. After enduring over a year of chemotherapy, he now had to decide whether to amputate, use a cadaver bone, or do nothing. Nothing was starting to sound pretty good.

Ashley and Skip had their usual discussion on the ride back to Charleston. Ashley couldn't believe what Skip had told her about the surgery. Even though it was Duke they were talking about, they both thought that, somehow, there must be a better alternative. A second opinion or some other resource must be available to them. Right then, Skip received a call from an old friend, George, whom he hadn't spoken to in years. They had spent summers together at the shore. In conversation it came up that Skip's friend was married now and his wife, Sarah, was an oncology nurse in the Washington, DC, area. Skip told George about his current health status; they both marveled at the coincidence of Sarah's working in not only oncology, but in orthopedic oncology. George thought it might be a good idea if Skip spoke directly with Sarah to see if she had any ideas on what to do next. It turns out that God was opening up new doors and putting the right people in Skip's life at the right time. Sarah told Skip that they were doing groundbreaking work on bone sarcomas at the Washington Hospital Center and the National Institute of Health in Washington, DC. She worked directly with the head of orthopedic oncology, Dr. Marvin Moore, who was at the helm of surgical advancement. Sarah had suggested that Ashley and Skip take a trip to DC to visit Dr. Moore and find out more about what techniques they were using for patients like Skip. Another answer to prayer. It all went back to the day the Duke pathologist diagnosed Skip, when Skip dropped to his knees and gave it all up to God to handle. Positive events kept happening.

†

The flight to Reagan National was uneventful. Although expensive, the flight was direct from Charleston to Washington, and in Skip's condition, it was worth every penny. Skip's parents, Mack and Maria, were still living in the suburbs of Washington and picked them up at the airport. The appointment with Dr. Moore was not until the following day. Mack drove up the George Washington Parkway and crossed over Key Bridge to take a shortcut to the Bethesda subdivision. They were living in the home that was originally built and bought by Mimi and Dominic. That house had now been in the family for more than fifty years. Skip was comforted upon his return to this residence, where he had nothing but fond memories. He and Ashley took the upstairs back bedroom, the room where Skip lived while attending graduate school and living with Mimi.

That night, they all decided to go to one of their favorite Italian restaurants, the Pines of Rome, which was just a couple of blocks away. It was inexpensive Italian cooking that was as close as one could get to what Maria or Mimi would make. Veal parmesan was the favorite for everyone.

Roast peppers were served on the side, with big jugs of Gallo wine to wash it down. The dinner was excellent and, as usual, no room for a cannoli.

✝

Mack woke Skip and Ashley early in order to get them down to the hospital center on time for their appointment. Skip slept well, but it was all relative because of the way he had to sleep on his back with his arm pain. It was too early for breakfast, so they decided to hit the road. Mack cut across East–West Highway and picked up New Hampshire Avenue that ran them straight down to the Washington Hospital Center. The ride from Bethesda was a little over thirty minutes without a lot of traffic. They passed Trinity College and Archbishop Carroll High School before turning right into the main parking area. Skip was filled with nervous anxiety as they approached the hospital.

The inside looked like a mini-Duke clinic. Although it had far fewer patients, it still possessed an aura of sadness. Skip and Ashley checked in at the desk and presented the requisite insurance information. It was 8:45 a.m., and their appointment was at 9:00 a.m. Skip wondered when he would actually be seen. He was armed like an attorney heading to court, with files of notes from Dr. Barker and x-rays and scans that had been taken back in Charleston. After about twenty minutes or so, Skip was called to the front and told that he needed to report to x-ray to have images taken of his arm area and his lungs.

Skip noticed a lot of younger kids in the other waiting rooms as he walked the halls from x-ray to his examination room. Ewing's sarcoma, after all, was generally an adolescent disease, with the majority of patients in their teens and younger.

Dr. Moore was a soft-spoken, diminutive man who walked in on Skip and Ashley in their waiting room with an entourage. Skip's friend Sarah was with him and greetings were exchanged all around. Dr. Moore examined Skip and ran him through a few physical tests to see what he could do with his arm. He was a colleague of Dr. Laurie at Duke and was well-versed in the techniques being used there. Dr. Moore agreed that the humerus bone should be replaced, although not with a cadaver bone. Dr. Moore and the team at the National Institute of Health had developed a titanium prosthesis that could be used in place of the cadaver bone. Until now, it had only been used by a handful of people, so there was not a lot of data on the prostheses.

Dr. Moore presented the bottom line to Skip and Ashley. He recommended having the surgery done by him at the Washington Hospital Center. The real kicker for Skip was that during the conversation with Dr. Moore, the doctor had mentioned the deleterious effects of the heavy doses of radiation that were applied to Skip's body. He also said that it was just a matter of time before that level of radiation led to another sarcoma in the arm. The only question was, would it be one year, ten years, or twenty years? Nobody knew. Taking out the radiated bone might prevent sarcoma from developing in the future.

Dr. Moore answered their questions and left them to think over the matter; he asked them to get back to him as soon as possible. The drive back to Bethesda was full of conversation and debate. One thing seemed unanimous: the cadaver replacement had just been taken off the list. As much as Skip liked Dr. Laurie, he couldn't bring himself to go that route. The only question that remained was whether or not to have the surgery. The doctors at all the institutions agreed that surgery was necessary in order to give Skip the best chance at beating the cancer. Skip was told before his chemotherapy at Duke that it would be an aggressive protocol that would take its toll on him. Although the warning was given, it really couldn't register with Skip who, at the time, knew nothing about chemo or its side effects. The situation with Dr. Moore was just the opposite. He didn't mention the severity of the surgery or the amount of time it would take to recover. Skip never really gave it a thought, but in hindsight he wished he had.

Maria had lunch waiting for them. It was really more like an early dinner, as they caught heavy traffic heading out of DC on the way back to Bethesda. Maria wanted to hear all about what was said and how her son was doing. The family discussed matters over an excellent meal of Maria's eggplant parmesan, salad, and bread. She had clearly inherited Mimi's cooking skills. Maria expressed her happiness at the tests being negative, but they had to decide what to do regarding the surgery, if anything. There really was no alternative. Skip needed the surgery, and they all knew it. He contacted Dr. Moore's office the next morning and conceded. With cancer, time is of the essence, so surgery was scheduled for two weeks later. This would barely give Skip and Ashley time enough to get home, get plans together for the kids, and get back up to DC.

✝

Back in Charleston, crispness penetrated the air. The Spanish moss hung on the live oak trees in the Sibleys' yard, swaying in the gentle breezes, as if to welcome them home. Fall in the Lowcountry again. It's unlike any other season. The oak trees hold tightly to their leaves, unwilling to relinquish them until spring. The grass remained bright green for an inordinate amount of time before going dormant for the season. The mussels and oysters were in season and could be harvested in the marsh behind the house. Skip and Caroline would go back there with her bucket and shovel, digging for black mussels in the vacant areas of pluff mud between the patches of spartina grass. They'd return with dozens of them that Caroline would proudly display to Ashley in the kitchen.

They decided it would be best if Ashley stayed at home with the kids during the initial surgery, and then later she would take them up to visit Skip during his recovery. Skip researched and found some organizations that helped those in need fly to hospitals around the country. He hooked up with Angel Flights and made arrangements with them to fly to DC for his cancer surgery. Although they did their best with regard to the patient's departure times and days, it was arranged on a standby, day-to-day basis. If Skip had to, he would catch a commercial flight at the last minute to get him there. Blessings were bestowed upon them, for Skip was able to catch one of the Angel Flights into Washington, where Mack and Maria would pick him up at Reagan National.

Skip spent his time during that two-week period at home with Ashley and the kids. He was regaining his strength as the chemo was wearing off. Thus, he had more energy to play with Foster and Caroline. They went up to the beach to look for shells and splashed around in the still-warm ocean water. The sea's saltwater rejuvenated Skip to an extent, and he experienced a peacefulness that can only come from looking out into a boundless ocean, the warm breeze on his skin. Skip had read that salt air was a natural healer, so he inhaled deeply as they strode up and down the beach.

Back at home, Ashley was preparing what she thought Skip might need for his surgical visit to DC. She knew that anything she overlooked would quickly be gotten by Mack and Maria. The two weeks passed quickly, and Skip was beginning to grow more anxious about his upcoming surgery. Did he really need it? Would everything turn out okay? Was there a chance that he might wake up out of surgery without an arm? The questions lingered. The closer it came time to leave, the more anxious was Skip. He became more solemn and distant with both Ashley and the kids. Fear of the unknown was upon him. After all, it was never really communicated to him what the procedure or the aftermath would be like. All Skip knew was that they were taking out a bad bone and putting in a metal rod. .

†

Angel Flights came through with a Gulfstream IV owned by a Fortune 500 company. It happened to be making a quick stop in Charleston before continuing on to Washington, DC. Skip said his good-byes on the tarmac of Charleston Airport. The plane took off from general aviation, meaning that one didn't have to actually go to the airport itself. General aviation was its own little microcosm, self-sustaining away from the masses. This allowed the Sibley family to escort Skip onto the plane without hassle. Not only was he flying for free, he was flying first class. Skip boarded the plane with arm in sling. His bag was checked by one of the crew. There were only four seats on the plane, and no passengers were on board except the two pilots in the front. Skip introduced himself and took a seat in the back row. Flying in a Gulf Stream jet is an awesome experience. If you have the means, it comes highly recommended. Moments later, two men in business attire boarded the plane and gave a cursory salute to the captain and then made their way back toward Skip. At this point, Skip was still bald, so they probably had an idea that he was a cancer patient. They became acquainted and exchanged stories. There appeared to be a sincere empathy from the businessmen and the pilots. Skip, in turn, learned that he was flying with the chief executive officer and the chief operating officer of a large firm. Skip exchanged Wall Street stories in an attempt to fit in with the high-powered moguls, and he thanked them repeatedly for the opportunity to fly with them and for all their hospitality. They were happy to help, exclaimed the CEO. The flight took off and both men and Skip were offered food by the co-pilot. A light lunch of sandwiches and beverages was passed around. Skip slowly removed himself from the conversation and let the men talk business for most of the remainder of the flight. He might have actually dozed off a time or two on the way. The flight from Charleston to Washington was a little over an hour and time passed very quickly. Before Skip knew it, the captain was signaling the passengers to fasten their seat belts and prepare for the descent into Reagan National. As the flight prepared to land, Skip caught a breathtaking view of the nation's capital. From the Washington Monument to the Capitol dome, he saw everything. He also saw what looked like the Masonic temple in Virginia off to his left. How magnificent. If only Skip were here to visit under different circumstances.

Skip was the only one disembarking in Washington. The businessmen had gone out of their way to take Skip to Washington on their way to Detroit. Skip thanked them again and went on his way into general aviation to find Mack and Maria.

✝

Ashley was home taking care of the usual business of working, raising the children, keeping up the house, and so forth. She had her hands full—

very full. The days merged together into one sleepless, exhausting day after another, and the routine was the same each day. Get up around 5:00 a.m. and get herself ready for work. Wake the children and get Caroline ready for school and Foster ready for day care. Caroline caught the bus to Whitesides Elementary School right in front of the house. Ashley would watch her walk down the driveway with Trovo following her each step of the way. Trovo would wait with her patiently until the bus came to pick her up. One down, one to go. Ashley would load little Foster and his things in the car and take him across town to the day care center, kiss him good-bye, and be on her way. Two down, work to go. Ashley, as previously mentioned, had a brutal commute of over an hour to her office each way. Just about everyone at work knew her situation and was sympathetic. Her boss was a girlfriend of hers and attempted to shield Ashley from any interaction with upper management. Her coworkers all had concern for her and her family. One, in particular, paid her a bit too much attention.

✝

Mack and Maria were thrilled to see Skip as he walked through the doors of the general aviation terminal. Skip told them that after flying in a Gulfstream, it would be difficult to squeeze back into a commercial coach flight. They were all in an upbeat mood as they made the trip back to Bethesda. Tomorrow was the big day, but little discussion took place about the surgery. Mack would take the day off, and he and Maria would take Skip down to the hospital. The surgery was scheduled for the crack of dawn, so they would be up and out early. Being back at the house on Maple Avenue brought back all kinds of memories and emotions for Skip. After all, he was raised there for a brief period as a young boy, and he also had those wonderful years living there with Mimi. After supper, the talk of the surgery began. Maria asked Skip and Mack just what was going to happen, but Skip knew little of what the next day would bring. He knew only that they were going to replace his right arm above the elbow and into the shoulder with a prosthetic device, eliminating the cancerous bone. What, Skip wondered aloud, did they do with the old bone once they examined it?

He thought of asking Dr. Moore if he could save it and give it to Trovo as a Christmas present. Bad idea. One critical thing Skip knew was that they were going to do a total biopsy of the bone to see if there was any cancer left in the arm pursuant to the radiation and chemotherapy.

Needless to say, sleep was difficult to come by that night. Skip couldn't stop thinking about the surgery, Ashley, and the kids at home. Was there a chance that he would not make it through the surgery, or that complications would require his arm being amputated during the procedure? If these scenarios were ever discussed, Skip certainly didn't remember them. He just wanted to be lying next to Ashley in their bed at home, tucking the children in for the night. He wasn't good with the weight of the world on his shoulders. Skip was an average guy going through a very unusual situation. How could he even think at this time that God might be using him in ways to further the kingdom and help others? Those thoughts never cross one's mind. One is too close to the situation and too concerned about the present to see the big picture. For a cancer patient, the future is now. There may be no tomorrow.

Only God knew when would be Skip's last breath on Earth. Skip was pleading that it wouldn't be tomorrow.

Chapter 11

POST-OP

†

"Do I still have my arm?" were Skip's first words upon awakening from surgery. Skip remembered nothing of the ten to twelve hours it took to replace his humerus bone. It was much, much more than he bargained for. The last thing Skip remembered was Dr. Moore and some of his surgical staff in a very cold, sterile operating room. Dr. Moore gave Skip a brief chat, mentioning that this was the hardest part for the surgeon, waiting for all the parts to come together so they can begin. It must be hospital protocol, but Dr. Moore double-checked with Skip that it was his "right" arm that they would be working on. Skip nodded in agreement, a blue mark was made on the arm, and the anesthesia was administered.

The highly specialized surgical team went to work. The prosthetic device was handmade especially for Skip. The job of the surgical team, led by Dr. Moore, was to replace the humerus bone with the prosthetic with as few complications as possible. The incision was some eighteen inches long, running from the top of the scapula down to almost the elbow. The skin was pulled back to expose the inner workings of the proximal portion of the arm. Muscle, tissue, tendons, and of course bone were all there waiting their turn to dance to the surgical orchestra. The tools used by Dr. Moore and his associates looked more like something you would find at Lowe's or Home Depot rather than at a hospital. Once the key muscles had been moved aside, only exposed bone remained. A device that resembled a small circular saw was used to cut the humerus bone just above the elbow at the bottom, and the bone was removed from its socket in the scapula at the top. At this point, the upper arm had essentially been amputated with the humerus bone now gone. Nurses used an array of instruments to keep the bleeding to a minimum. While Dr. Moore was busy with the patient, other doctors were readying the prosthetic device for implantation. Going back to his "Home Depot" toolbox, Dr. Moore drilled a long, deep hole in Skip's right elbow. This would be the place where the prosthetic device would be inserted. The device was long and protruding and had a two-to-three inch titanium dowel rod attached to the bottom that would be cemented into the newly drilled hole. It was meant to secure the bottom of the prosthesis to the elbow. The top of the device looked almost like a microphone, with a large ball that would fit into the socket of the shoulder. To this day, Skip is still not sure how this portion of the prosthesis is held in place. He thought he heard duct tape and super glue but wasn't sure.

Skip was sewn up and wheeled to intensive care to be monitored post-op. Again, Skip remembered none of this. As a matter of fact, he was not sure what he remembered when first regaining consciousness.

†

Mack and Maria spoke with Dr. Moore after the operation. They should have joined the hospital meal plan because they were there for breakfast, lunch, and dinner. Dr. Moore, in his surgical garb, relayed the good news that all went well with the surgery. The prosthesis was in place and, just as important, there were no additional signs of cancer in the remaining bone. Maria gave Dr. Moore a big hug, and Mack thanked him profusely. Maria called Ashley on the house phone but, to her surprise, Ms. Janie picked up and said that she was glad to hear Skip was doing well. Ashley was still at work. Ms. Janie told Maria that she and her church were sending up prayers all day for Skip and his healing. Maria thought that it was a little peculiar that Ashley was working at eight o'clock in the evening and assumed she was still getting situated with her new position. Maria said good-bye to Ms. Janie and asked her to have Ashley call them as soon as possible.

✝

What just happened? A woman was tugging on Skip trying to get him to do something. Pain. "There must be some mistake," Skip thought in his semiconscious state. There was nothing but pain. On a scale from one to ten, his pain was a twelve. He was slowly beginning to realize that he was in a hospital bed in a room with all kinds of contraptions hooked up to him. He was originally fitted with a morphine drip, but apparently during the night he couldn't handle it and was throwing up all over himself, so the nurses turned off the morphine. It was morning now, or so Skip thought. What was all this about? It was coming back to him very slowly. The drugs and the pain made it difficult to concentrate. The nurse kept pestering him, and he kept ignoring her, but not on purpose. Skip had been taken from intensive care during the night to a private room early the following morning. Mack and Maria went home after they heard the news the previous evening and would return at some point that morning.

Skip noticed that his right arm was elevated and was bandaged beyond recognition. Was this the source of his torment? It was coming back to him in slow drips. Cancer. He had cancer and was having an operation. The pain continued. Skip did not consciously think it, but Jesus must be close, because those who suffer are drawn close to the Lord. "Someone please help me," Skip cried. "God help me," he moaned before being pronged by the nurse again. Apparently, it was time for Skip to have his first post-op x-ray to see what the arm looked like after the prosthesis had been inserted. How could he possibly move out of the bed? There was no way that he could physically make this happen. The nurse was belligerent with Skip in her vain attempts to move him from the bed. She even used profanity in an attempt to get him up. Skip began to yell and scream for Dr. Moore. He needed help. He needed pain medicine badly. Skip demanded that he see a doctor to know why he must be moved in his current state. The cantankerous nurse finally acquiesced and left the room for additional help. Skip was so out of it and had so many drugs in his system that he just broke down and cried, trying to figure things out. By the time the next person entered the room, Skip had regained a little control of himself, but he could not believe what he was experiencing. The new nurse calmly explained to Skip that they needed to wheel him down to X-Ray to take a few pictures of his new arm. Knowing it was one thing, but actually getting out of the bed and into the wheelchair was another. It took both nurses and several orderlies to move Skip from his bed to a wheelchair. Skip needed the wheelchair to travel. It was never mentioned to him that it would be several weeks before he might be able to walk again. How could surgery on the arm affect the ability to walk? These and other thoughts crisscrossed through Skip's mind as the process was unfolding.

The images were remarkable, and the radiologist asked Skip if he wanted to take a look at his new arm. It looked like a microphone with it being narrow at the bottom and long and bulbous at the proximal portion. Once he had seen the image, Skip wanted to be put back in his bed.

✝

It was still early in the morning when Mack got the call from Ashley about the surgery. She apologized for not getting back to them the night of the surgery, but she didn't get home until late that evening and didn't want to wake Mack and Maria. Ashley was relieved to hear of the news that the cancer had not spread further and that Skip was out of intensive care. Mack told her that he was in immense pain, and they were trying to figure out how to put him a little more at ease. Everything was done in the hospital bed, including bowel movements, which made Skip wonder how anyone could be a nurse. He was hooked up at both ends—or so he thought—and they were changed on a regular basis.

✝

The hospital experience was one that Skip couldn't have predicted. It was a complete and total nightmare. No one had warned him of this post-op mayhem or explained how he was going to feel after the surgery. Skip had serious regrets at this point about having the procedure done. "Could it be worth the pain?" he would cry out to God. God was silent, but the emotions of perseverance kept taking hold. Just when he thought he was finished dancing through the nightmare of chemotherapy, he was thrust into this major surgery. In retrospect, he should have asked more questions and should have assumed that having his arm cut off for a certain amount of time would be painful. The procedure aside, the hospital center was the world's worst place that Skip had ever been. From getting a hold of a doctor or a nurse, to the food and general treatment, it was all intolerable. Skip was an easygoing guy and wasn't one who liked to make a lot of waves when he didn't like something. He was more apt to just stay quiet and hope that things would get better.

He was visited briefly by his parents on the first day after surgery. They were vocal advocates for Skip in getting him the things that he needed. They found it just as frustrating as Skip to get anything meaningful done. Getting a nurse took forever. Any pain medication was always questioned. Skip would respond with, "Hello, I just had my arm cut off; I would like a little something for the pain, thank you." The hospital was mismanaged and understaffed. The general lack of concern for the patient was disturbing. Mack told Skip that *U.S. News & World Report* had just ranked this place as one of the ten best hospitals in America. If that were so, Skip pitied the other 99 percent of hospitals in America. Some of the best and brightest doctors around, like Dr. Moore, had privileges at the hospital, which is probably why it was ranked so highly.

Skip was in the hospital for almost two weeks, with one day being as agonizing as the next. One of the first days after the surgery, a young female physical therapist came by his room to tell him it was time for his therapy.

Skip was less than forty-eight hours out of surgery when the attempt was made to get him to do something physical. Skip was mortified that he might have to do anything except crawl back under the covers and make this girl go away. "The quicker you start rehabilitating, the quicker and easier it will become," she told him. Skip envisioned her making him do curls with a dumbbell or one-arm pushups, but all she wanted this first day was for him to walk. Get him to walk! Until he tried, Skip realized that he was unable to walk under his own power. How could this be? The surgery was to his arm. Apparently, the magnitude of the surgery was so severe that it was a total shock to all parts of Skip's body. The process of sitting up in bed, getting down on his feet, and with the aid of the physical therapist holding him, walking to the door and back took almost an hour. When Skip got back in the bed, he jokingly replied to the nurse, "Man, am I out of shape." This routine went on daily, with distances increasing each day until Skip was able, still with the aid of the therapist, to walk to the end of the hallway and back to his room. No attempt was made to rehab the arm. Skip needed to get his strength back first.

✝

Other than Mack and Maria visiting him each day, Skip had no other visitors. Just like being in the hospital during chemotherapy, he didn't feel like talking and really didn't want to see anyone anyway. Skip was still in a battle with the hospital staff over pain relief. He couldn't sleep at night, and he was in acute pain most of the day. He really just wanted someone to hit him over the head with a hammer and wake him up when it was time to go home. Out of the blue one afternoon, a college friend of Skip's who lived in Virginia stopped by the hospital to visit him. Bruce Palmer and Skip were fraternity brothers at the Phi Delta Theta house at Gettysburg College in the early '80s. Bruce and Skip had stayed in pretty close contact over the years, close enough that he would come by the hospital to check on Skip.

The devil was tormenting Skip this particular day. Before Bruce showed up, Skip was in pain and could get no relief. He was talking to himself and yelling at no one in particular. Was the devil making him suffer so? Was this an attempt to draw Skip farther from God? All Bruce knew was that when he walked in the room that afternoon, Skip was yelling and crying about nothing in particular. Bruce tried to hold a rational, nonpsychotic conversation with Skip, who was unable to participate from his point of view. He just kept yelling for the nurse and crying to Bruce to help him because he was in such pain. Bruce, being a mild-mannered sort, called for a nurse for Skip but, as usual, there was no one around to help. Bruce decided that he wasn't doing Skip any help by being there, so he said good-bye and went on his way. Years later the two hooked up again with their families to take in a Washington Nationals baseball game at the old Robert F. Kennedy Stadium. Somehow in conversation, that visit Bruce made to the hospital years ago came up. As Bruce had thought, Skip had no recollection of Bruce ever being there. The Nationals lost to the Braves that evening by a score of three to one.

✝

The days at the hospital merged together. Skip doesn't remember, but Dr. Moore came by several times during his rounds to check on Skip. After all, there were less than two dozen of these types of procedures done worldwide to date, so the doctor had a keen interest in Skip's progress. Skip was told on one of his post-op office visits that he would be one of the star patients in Dr. Moore's new book on limb salvaging surgery, no doubt a *New York Times* best seller and a must-read for the two dozen patients and their doctors.

Rehab was going poorly. Skip fought it every step of the way. He wanted no part of any additional pain that might come from the therapy. He missed the bigger picture that this would probably make him feel better sooner if he just listened to the therapist. Mack and Maria were real advocates for Skip. Without them, it would be a miracle if they even realized he was in his room half the time. Nowadays, patients must have someone with them at a medical facility to act as a voice or advocate for the patient. Usually the patient is the last one to remember to do something, and everything is so difficult. An advocate, whether it's a family member or a friend, can keep the staff in line better and helps the patient get what he or she needs.

One morning before Mack and Maria arrived, one of the employees was emptying the trash can in Skip's bathroom. Moments later that same employee was at Skip's bedside to draw blood! Budget cuts must have been in full effect at this place. Skip, being a mild-mannered guy, just assumed that the lady emptying the trash can washed her hands before taking his blood.

There was a celestial battle being waged in Skip's head, and the demons were winning. The pain and suffering continued throughout his stay at the hospital. Skip cast out these demons in the name of Jesus. He knew that Jesus was near those who were sick and suffering. Just as Job of the Bible was cursed by Satan, Skip painted an image of an epic battle between God and Satan as to who would get his soul. The evil one walks among us and causes us much grief in this life. Do not fall for it, because only God can save a person for all eternity. God brought Job to his knees with earth-shattering pain and suffering, but Job never lost his faith in God. Conditions were hard, but Skip held on to this strength that God gave Job in his transcendent battle.

✝

It was discharge time, and not a moment too soon. Skip would rank this hospital stay right up there with the worst of the chemotherapy hospital visits. The two were starkly different in all aspects, but pain and suffering were the common denominator, just in a different form. The pain from the chemo was not so much a physical pain as it was an overall body malfunction. Everything felt wrong, from his stomach to his head and all that was in between. It was a slow, torturous journey during each weekly visit, where Skip had come to know what was coming his way and how it was going to make him feel. There was always a wistful yearning that chemo week would come to an end quicker, although it never did.

The surgery blindsided Skip, and he never really recovered from that hospital encounter. He was woefully unprepared for the dealings that had come his way. Who could know what to expect after having an arm amputated and a prosthetic limb put in its place? Nevertheless, the horribleness of the hospital visit had finally come to an end, and Mack and Maria were there to take him home. As customary, a wheelchair was summonsed to cart Skip out of the hospital. Most of the time, this was hospital protocol, but in this event, Skip still did not have his sea legs and was in need of the wheelchair. Skip mumbled a quick good-bye and good riddance as he was pushed to the outside light for the first time in several weeks. It was good to be out of the hospital and going home.

It was a struggle getting Skip from the car to the Maple Avenue house. Mack did his best to help Skip, who had lain down for most of the ride home from the hospital. The arm was very, very fragile and his pain considerable. A couch was set up on the first floor of the den close to the rear entrance. This would give Skip a temporary place to lie until he had the strength to go up the stairs to his old back bedroom. Orders written for Skip by Dr. Moore at the hospital included arm elevation. Once Skip got in a somewhat comfortable position on the couch, Mack thought he would attempt to elevate Skip's arm and place some pillows underneath. Maria stood there and gasped as Mack yanked Skip's arm up about a foot and put the pillows underneath. A viral scream was all that was heard for the next few minutes, as Skip could not breathe from the encounter and was in so much pain that he cried in mercy. His eyes again were as wide as saucers. Mack, meaning no harm, did not have a nurse's touch when elevating the arm. That is the most Skip's arm had moved vertically since he underwent the surgery. Maria went to the kitchen for pain medicine, all the while yelling at Mack to be more careful.

†

Now that Skip was out of the hospital, Ashley was planning a trip up with the kids. Things were going well at home. Ms. Janie was still coming to help out several times a week, as Ashley was spending more time at work. Caroline and Foster loved Ms. Janie; she would tell them stories and take them on walks in the neighborhood. Ashley was placed on a team with several other employees to work on a computer project that was vital to her department. As many coworkers do, they often went out to lunch together and occasionally bonded at an after-work happy hour.

Ashley had little leave or vacation time left, so it was difficult to get away for an extended period. The company had a leave fund whereby those retiring with extra leave could donate that leave to a leave bank for other employees to use. Ashley applied for several days out of that bank for her trip with the kids to go up to DC to see Skip. The bank was a blessing, as it let Ashley stay for a little over a week. They would leave tomorrow and be in DC to see their long-missed daddy.

✝

The transition from hospital to home was a welcome one, although the patient was still seriously ill. Recovery would not be quick or smooth by any means. After several days of staying in the downstairs den, Skip felt up for moving upstairs to his old bedroom in the rear of the second floor above the den addition. Still too weak to walk on his own, he could only get up and down the stairs with the help of Mack. The bedroom was small but comfortable and was Skip's own private oasis were he could be alone with his thoughts. The room held many memories for Skip. It originally hosted his Uncle Donnie, who utilized the bedroom during his college days at Montgomery Junior College and later the University of Maryland. Donnie hadn't set a land speed record for leaving the house. His eight years of college were wearing thin on Poppop, who of course was footing the bill. Poppop used to tell Donnie that he'd better graduate with a medical degree for being in school so long.

There was also a period when Jacqueline inherited the room. Skip was foggy on when and why this was but was certain that she spent time there. And then there were the raucous days of Skip's graduate school years when he assumed control over the room. It served as both a bedroom and study area. Skip set up an old card table on which to do his work, one that was probably used by Poppop or Donnie to play poker years before. Modest accommodation by most standards, this room was just what Skip needed. And the price was right—free!

The first few days at the house Skip had tried to get a handle on his medication. It was only two weeks post-op, and Dr. Moore's staff was suggesting that he take Advil or Tylenol for the pain. No, this would not do. Once again, an advocate was needed, and Maria was the perfect candidate. She was relentless with the hospital and the doctor's staff on getting Skip the pain medicine that he so desperately needed. This seemed like an endless tug of war, where one almost had to beg to get anything from the doctors. Skip could understand their concern about addiction to pain medication, but he was still in such pain that Advil wasn't going to cut it. Short-duration prescriptions were subscribed, and when they ran out, Maria would venture through the whole process over and over again.

With the night came discomfort and terror. Sleep was impossible. Skip couldn't find a comfortable position in which his arm stayed elevated. Nighttime was also Satan's time. The drugs were playing with his mind and his state of mental health. Depression was knocking on the door, constantly present to battle with his inner thoughts. He heard voices and saw shadowy outlines. He was even visited by Jacqueline one night. She spoke but was not seen, but Skip felt the presence of someone in the room with him. More voices. Skip did not speak. Jacqueline had come to tell Skip that there was indeed a heaven; yet, her voice was melancholy as she revealed this information. Jackie never mentioned where she was, but Skip believed that heaven had eluded her, and she was in another place—not hell, but somewhere else. Satan was playing tricks on Skip, testing him as he did Jesus in the wilderness. There were many times when Skip thought of giving up on life, but they revolved around the pain and suffering of the cancer and the chemotherapy. This was different. It was as if Jackie was being used by Satan to communicate to Skip the ultimate lie that heaven will evade him perhaps as well. The room was cold, and Skip attempted to cast out what he thought were demons in the name of Jesus. The room was at peace for the moment, so Skip dozed off.

It was morning. Skip's first thoughts revolved around the pain of sleep, but then he remembered what happened the night before. Was it real? Did it really happen? He let it slip from his mind for a time, as Maria came in the room to check on him and to see if he wanted any breakfast. Mack was working this day, so Skip would be confined to his quarters upstairs until evening. With the daylight came hope that so eluded him last night during his encounter with his sister.

✝

The one thing that the hospital and the doctor's office were on top of was inflicting more pain upon the patient. Skip had been home two days when he was paid a visit by the occupational therapist. It was time to start getting the arm better. Skip was reticent about having someone come to the house for therapy, but on the upside, he wouldn't have to leave the house. The therapist was young and pleasant and showed Skip a written schedule they'd follow to get his basic motor skills functioning. The therapy was something a child could do, but it was of the utmost difficulty for Skip. Merely putting his arm on the table and reaching out was a monumental task. The idea was to see whether his hand and fine motor skills were working. Initially there was very little movement in the hand, but as the therapy sessions continued, so did the progress. Skip would regain the use, for the most part, of the fine motor skills of his right hand, although this would take some time. The therapist spent about an hour with Skip three times a week. This schedule would continue for a while.

✝

Mack was home from work and asked Skip if he wanted to come down for dinner and stay downstairs for a while and watch the Yankees and Mets World Series. Skip was definitely up for time away from the upstairs room. Home cooking was a pleasure beyond belief for Skip as he devoured Maria's homemade sauce and spaghetti. Everything at this point was obviously done left-handed. Skip didn't realize that for most functions in life going forward, he would be a lefty for good. Skip ate very slowly as he was adjusting to eating with his left hand. Basic, everyday skills that one takes for granted were no longer easy for Skip. Everything was a struggle.

Mack helped Skip from the table and walked him into the family room. Skip positioned himself on the couch with Mack and Maria taking the armchairs. Maria reminded Skip that Ashley and the kids would be here in the morning. Skip had not entirely forgotten this, but it was a good reminder. He knew they were coming; he just wasn't exactly sure when. He couldn't wait to see Ashley and especially the kids. It had been several weeks since he'd seen the family and was looking forward to some hugs and kisses.

The game was good with the Yankees beating the Mets four to one in game one of the series. Skip managed to stay awake for the most part, dozing in and out several times during the final innings. Afterward, Mack carried Skip up the stairs to the back room for another night of rest.

She appeared quickly on this evening. The room again grew cold and Skip thought he heard the blinds and curtains moving. With the door shut, it was very dark in the room, with only a limited glow reflecting through one of the windows from an outside porch light. The thought of calling out for Mack or Maria never occurred to Skip. He sat in the bed alone with his thoughts and questions. Detaching himself from reality was not hard, with all of the drugs he had taken before bed. Unlike the apparitions experienced by Ashley, there was no sense of peace in the room, only uncertainty and fear. The hair rose on the back of Skip's neck as he saw what he believed to be an outline of the figure of Jacqueline standing next to the bed. Skip spoke to her, but she did not respond. She only hovered for what seemed like an eternity before she spoke. The apparition was blurred, so Skip could not see well as Jacqueline moved closer. "There is a heaven, and it is a wonderful place," she said. Her voice still had a ring of sorrow as she spoke almost the same words again: "Heaven is real, and it is a wonderful place." The room remained cool as Jackie disappeared again. This would be the last time she would present herself to Skip. Laying in a cold sweat and wondering what had just happened, Skip momentarily came back to his senses. Jackie had been dead for some twenty years. Why would she pick this time and place to show herself to him? Skip had a dreadful feeling that somehow Jackie did in fact have a taste of heaven, but she wasn't actually there. Surely she couldn't be in hell. This was a place for those who turned their backs on God and rejected Jesus during their lifetimes. But Jackie did not fit this mold. She was young and was raised in the church. Still, nobody could really know someone else's heart. Skip would lament these thoughts and fall back on fond memories of Jacqueline during their youth. But why was the room so cold? Why wouldn't she talk to Skip more about heaven and transcendental life?

✝

The room was warm. This was the day that Ashley and the children would be arriving. What a night. Skip decided he wouldn't mention to Mack and Maria the apparitions of Jacqueline the past two evenings, as he thought it might upset them, or that something was wrong with him. But something *was* wrong with him. He still had cancer and was seeing visions of his sister who had been dead for more than twenty years. His mental health was unstable at best, but he couldn't realize it. He was right in the middle of it or looking down on it from the outside. How could he understand what was going on when he was fighting for his life? Coping with everyday life was a struggle, to say the least. Pain, confusion, visions, life and death, not seeing his family all took a toll on him. Skip didn't know how to ask for help in this regard, and no one around him was able to fully grasp his situation. The cancer was out in the open, but the remainder of the unsightliness stayed hidden. Skip was simply tucking away these thoughts and feelings. He could deal with only so much at once. It would one day come to the surface.

Chapter 12
AN AFFAIR

✝

She said she would be leaving tomorrow for a week or so to visit Skip after his surgery. Bob took it all in stride, as the good Christian had maneuvered his way into another woman's life. Bob was a predator who patrolled the waters for women in need. Whether it was a bad marriage, financial difficulties, strife at work, whatever, Bob was there to pick up their pieces. Ashley fit the bill to a tee. The sex was the trophy begotten by Bob for his conquests.

It was late and Ashley had a lot to do to prepare to leave with the kids in the morning. Bob suggested a "quickie" in Ashley's car. Presently, Ashley was committed, so the rendezvous took place without a hitch. For Bob, one man's pleasure was another man's pain.

✝

Skip's third night home from the hospital was a terrible one. The dichotomy of his dream to real life was haunting. His fragility was met in his dreams with violence. In one particular dream, Skip was brutally thrown around his room like a rag doll. He cried out to God to stop as he was about to be thrown down the stairs in this vile nightmare. Skip was actually vocalizing his torment, which brought Mack and Maria into the room to check on him. He was soaked in a cold sweat and crying for the nightmare to stop. Maria held him and told him that he was just having a bad dream, and that everything would be okay. But the coldness in the room was still present as it had been when Jackie appeared. The demons were near and were causing Skip distress. He told his parents about the dream and the cold and the devil, but they assured him he was just having a bad dream. Perhaps the pain medicine was causing these hallucinations. Skip didn't want any more medicine at the time. Since it was the middle of the night and he couldn't go back to sleep, he cut on the television for some background noise to keep the demons at bay.

✝

Skip was surrounded by familiar faces. Mack had gotten up early to head out to Reagan National to pick up Ashley and the kids. What a welcomed sight. Skip couldn't stop kissing the children, and Ashley looked as beautiful as ever. They planned on staying four or five days. Ashley got the time off from work. Caroline could miss a little school, and Foster had no place he'd rather be. Skip came down for breakfast, and they all caught up on what's been going on at home. Ashley told Skip that all the neighbors sent their best and couldn't wait to see him around the neighborhood. For some reason, David Gorham had Ashley bring Skip a cigar. Knowing that Skip didn't smoke—and it was probably the worst thing for someone going through cancer—David said it would make Skip laugh and remind him of home and the good ol' times. That it did.

It just so happened that their visit coincided with Halloween—needless to say an important night in the lives of the young children. The Teletubbies were a big hit, so Foster went trick-or-treating as Po, the smallest and red

Teletubbie. Caroline in true fashion went as a fairy princess. Ashley and the proud grandparents walked the children from house to house in the suburban Bethesda neighborhood of Lynbrook. Skip, though, was unable to make the rounds, so he stayed home and manned the front door for the little ghouls and goblins that might come knocking. It was actually the last thing Skip felt like doing, so he politely placed a bowl of candy with his left arm on the front porch and, like any good agoraphobic, turned the porch light out and went into the back den to watch the World Series. It wasn't long before the gang returned with plenty of treats to last the duration of the trip.

Skip and Mack caught Ashley up on the latest progress and news on Skip and the arm. They ran the gamut from trying to get pain medication from the doctors to the occupational therapy visits. All in all, though, it was still the pain that kept Skip down. He had more steel in him by way of staples holding his arm together than the USS Yorktown. A nurse would also visit Skip a couple times a week to check his wounds and change his bandages and so on. As it was still very hard to walk on his own, Skip relied on Mack for his every move and was basically house ridden.

With the family in town, time moved quickly. Too quickly. It would still be several weeks before Skip would make the journey back to Charleston. Mack and Maria were already arranging another Angel Flight for Skip to take home. It was just so much more comfortable and easy to use the Angel Flight. Skip didn't know if he was even capable of maneuvering through the ins and outs of a commercial flight. His fragile arm made his ability to fly all the more uncertain. Angel Flights did not operate on a regular basis, so when they called and offered something, one had to be ready to pick up and go.

Skip and Maria said good-bye to Ashley and the children as it was time to hit the road to catch their flight back to Charleston. Ashley gave Skip a peck on the check and said she would see him in a couple of weeks. Mack had the route down pat by this time. He was better than a chauffeur and didn't mind the ride downtown. It was a scenic route that allowed views of all of the monument grounds, circling behind the Kennedy Center and Lincoln Memorial, while heading over the 14th Street Bridge into Virginia. Arlington National Cemetery could be seen at the top of the hill as one crossed from the district into Virginia. Mack pulled in front of the USAir departure terminal and unloaded the luggage for the group. A valet checked their bags curb side. Hugs and kisses went all around and, after the good-byes, they were off.

✝

The nurse was visiting that morning and was going to remove the staples. Skip wasn't quite sure what was holding his bandaged arm in place, but he assumed it was something significant. The nurse wanted Maria to observe the removal so she could teach her how to take care of the wound each day. The nurse began by taking the bandages off ever so carefully as not to hurt Skip. She told him this would hurt more than taking the staples out, but Skip highly doubted that. The bandages were about off, and the nurse called Maria over for a look. The next thing he knew, Maria had fallen to the floor in a fainting spell after one look at Skip's arm. The nurse revived her and got her a cold compress for her head, but said that she still needed to witness the removal of the staples and learn the cleaning methods. It was one of the most horrific sights for Maria as far as injuries go. From the elbow to the scapula, nothing but staples held the skin in place to heal after the surgery. Maria moved slowly back and forth from looking to not looking as the nurse removed the staples one by one. As Skip had thought, this was a little more painful than removing the bandages. The entire process took what seemed like hours, but was actually only about fifteen minutes. Once the staples were out, the nurse showed Maria how to care for the wound. Maria told the nurse that she wasn't sure if she could handle this on a regular basis, but the nurse assured her that it would heal and get better every day. Reluctantly, Maria agreed to assume the task, knowing that Mack would be there if she needed a helping hand.

The nurse was right; after the first several days, the task of cleaning and even just looking at the arm became easier for Maria. Maria had a handle on the situation and wasn't in need of any help from Mack. After Mack's first endeavor of lifting Skip's arm on day one, it was better that he was not involved. He really didn't understand pain thresholds because he had never really been a patient of any kind in his life. Mack would have made a horrible nurse.

The phone rang, and it was Angel Flights saying they had an available space in two days to Charleston if Skip wanted to take it. The timing was good, and Skip was starting to feel a little better, so they made the arrangements. If it was anything like the trip up to Bethesda, Skip would be able to handle the flight back to Charleston.

The surgery and this part of the ordeal were over. It seemed like a different life from the time he flew up till now. So much had happened in so little time. Skip was woefully unprepared for the surgery and aftermath. It was much more than he bargained for. And it really was only the beginning. The post-op therapy and rehabilitation could take anywhere from six months to a year. At this point, Skip had no use of the arm, and everything was done with the left hand or with the help of others.

Mack and Maria loaded the car with Skip's belongings and headed yet again to the airport. This was a bittersweet good-bye because of all they had been through together. It's not every day one's adult son goes through major cancer surgery and begins his recuperation at his parents' house. Mack assured Skip that if he needed anything, they would be the first to help. Maria mentioned coming down to watch the kids and lend a helping hand if she could.

General aviation was bustling in the nation's capitol. They found the Learjet, undoubtedly owned by some large corporation, and they said their good-byes. Skip was in much worse shape on the way back than he was on the way up, so he avoided conversation with the other guests and spent his entire trip sleeping in the rear seat. Then, the captain signaled their approach into Charleston, and he told everyone to fasten their seat belts. Skip felt a rush of exhausting excitement to be back home. But it wouldn't last.

Chapter 13

GRIEF

†

Skip hugged Ashley at the airport. He was tearful from the long, arduous process that he had been dealing with. Ashley seemed no worse for the wear and hugged Skip as well. The kids were back at the house being watched by one of the neighbors. Ashley told Skip that they couldn't wait to see their daddy today. The Angel Flight went well. One look at Skip and Ashley knew that there was no way he could have flown on a commercial jet. The ride from the airport to Bay Club was about half an hour. For all that was going on in each of their lives, they spoke little during the drive. Skip had taken some medicine at the airport, which made him less inclined to converse, but the usually gregarious Ashley seemed focused on something else.

†

The night before Skip arrived home, Ashley was catching up on some work at the office before making the long drive back to Charleston when Bob stopped by her desk to see how she was doing. He pulled up a chair, although uninvited, and asked Ashley if she wanted to grab a bite to eat. Ashley had so much going on with the kids and Skip's return the following day that she really needed to head home. She said she would take a rain check and see him at the office tomorrow.

✝

The door opened and Skip was mauled by what seemed like an army, but it was only Foster, Caroline, and Trovo. Trovo hadn't seen his master in a long time, but dogs never forget; he was ready to play ball as soon as Skip walked in. Caroline had made artwork that was a magnet for the refrigerator and was very proud to show it off to Daddy. Foster was excited as well, trying to squeeze his way in between Caroline, Trovo, and Ashley. Skip could not lift him but gave him a great big hug and kiss.

David Gorham had seen the car pull into the driveway and came over to check on his boy. The two hugged and caught up on events in each other's lives over the last month or so. David said the neighborhood had been dead since Skip had been gone. Skip knew he was just kidding as Skip rarely ventured from the confines of his house. Still, it was good to be home.

✝

Emotions ran deep as the lunchtime rendezvous at the nearby Holiday Inn came to an end. Bob had worked his magic on Ashley again, and they had just ended another episode in their sordid affair. There is usually no shortage of badmouthing the other partner, so Bob was quick to tell Ashley that Skip didn't love her or have the same feelings for her that he did. Given Ashley's state of mind, the mental and physical exhaustion made her easy prey and wide open to accept his rhetoric. She didn't want to believe him but continued carrying on this furtive relationship for many months to come. Skip, the children, the future of the family—did any of this cross her mind while she was committing adultery? People have a way of rationalizing the choices they make, and this apparently was no exception. Ashley needed comfort and love that she felt she wasn't or couldn't get from Skip at home, so Bob filled the void with his cacophony of nonsense. Ashley was hooked and she knew it, but she did nothing about it. She was, however, able to turn the switch on at work and off at home, with no change in her demeanor or countenance at home with Skip and the children. She wanted to end it quickly and look on it as the huge mistake it was, but with Bob always on the prowl, the situation could not be stopped. Try as she might, the overwhelming urges took her over, and she relinquished time and time again. All the while, Skip was home nursing his cancer and arm either alone, or with Ms. Janie, who was back to help now that Skip had returned. Ashley's having an adulterous affair was the farthest thing from Skip's mind.

✝

Skip had started his new routine at home: a combination of physical therapy and spending time with the kids. He was still in horrible shape, and it was still very difficult to walk. His strength was severely diminished, and he remained on the painkillers for relief from the constant aching of the arm. The occupational therapist in Charleston was coming to the house two to three times a week to help Skip get some of his hand and arm motion back. Skip could barely feed himself, could not dress himself, and was dependent on someone else for just about every aspect of his life. Caroline helped him get dressed some mornings by putting his belt on, or helping him tie his shoes. But all his basic motor skills were gone. He was relearning everything, and mostly from the left-hand side.

Although he was not yet up for attending church, Skip was reading a daily devotional given to him by David Gorham. It was good for his mind and faith. Skip never questioned why this happened to him and his family, and his faith in God was now strong. Skip was at the point where his conversations with Ms. Janie, Gorham, and others were really sinking in. Skip had become a believer. God could have taken him with the cancer, but he let him live. There must be a reason for his being here, and it would become his quest to find that reason and fulfill it for God.

✝

Ashley and Bob were in full swing in their romantic adventures. What began as a one-time fling had grown into somewhat of a relationship, according to Ashley. The Holiday Inn near their office was the location of choice, and it became a place of frequent encounters. Bob tried to talk Ashley into leaving Skip, telling her lies that the situation at home would be an endless struggle, and besides, Skip didn't love her anyway. Lies and more lies filled her head as her sultriness led her further and further into his web. She would go with the flow for the time being, somehow putting it out of her mind and spirit as she attempted to resume a normal life at home with Skip and the kids. Skip attributed the late nights and overworking to her new position at the firm. After all, they needed the benefits that the company was offering, like health insurance and sick leave. Skip's operation alone was close to $100,000 when all was said and done. He couldn't imagine where they would be without the health insurance of Ashley's employer. Once they reached their out-of-pocket maximum, which was a paltry $2,000, the rest was covered by the insurance company. Skip was an insurance company's worst nightmare. Living with cancer and going through radiation, chemotherapy, and an expensive surgery were not what the actuaries generally factored into their forecasts.

Skip's income took a hit as well. He obviously was not able to work between the time of onset through the surgery, and his last job left him with no source of ongoing funds. Skip was a gracious recipient of federal social security disability income. The only problem was it took six months to kick in. Well, not really the only problem. The amount was barely enough for the family to survive on, along with what Ashley was making. God gave them just what they could handle at this point and provided enough money to make it through each day. How ironic, living in a "mansion," as Caroline would call it on social security income. Money was tight, and with two kids and Ms. Janie, daily life was downright expensive. Again, God is good and met their needs during these trying times. Skip wasn't sure what Ashley was paying Ms. Janie, but he knew it wasn't enough to cover what she was doing. Her therapy sessions alone on the open market would cost Skip $100 an hour. It was all worth it for her sweet potato pies, though.

Skip didn't realize it, but he was suffering from depression, like a lot of cancer survivors do.

The fear and anxiety alone were enough to send you off the deep end, always wondering when and if it will be your turn to go. Does God have plans for me here on Earth, or is it my time to go to heaven? Why do some get to stay and some get to go? Skip had already lost several close friends to cancer along his journey, yet he remains. Why? It was simple: he had not yet fulfilled the task for which God put him on Earth. And the others had fulfilled their task? The pastor's wife with young children who died of breast cancer, had she already fulfilled her mission in life according to God? It had to be that way, Skip determined, or why else would such things happen. To those of us who remain, we grieve for those gone, and wonder why they were taken. We must remember that our time on this rock is so short compared to eternity, that doing God's will on Earth is what we are here to do. Those who believe in Jesus will have eternity to spend together, so we should not be so contemptuous of death on this sinned planet. Only you and God know in your heart whether you truly believe in him and wish to be with him for eternity. For hell is nothing more than the separation of you from God for eternity. What could be worse? Skip's depression and drug-induced pain relief were turning him into a modern-day theologian. But really, nothing else mattered. Skip would tell Caroline that as long as they both believed in God, nothing could ever separate them. We all suffer to some degree in this broken world, but the ultimate goal awaits us one day when we are called home. Skip was to find out shortly that his suffering had only just begun.

Ashley flew up the stairs to find Skip in the bathroom with the kids. She looked winded. Skip figured she'd had a tough day. He didn't figure on what would come next.

✝

Ms. Janie was still downstairs and about to put the kids to bed after their bath. She never really said good-bye, but kind of came and went like the wind. Once the coast was clear, Ashley returned to Skip with a puzzling look on her face. Not remorseful, though, for what she was about to lay on good ol' Skip. Ashley asked Skip if he had gotten a phone call from a woman tonight.

"No, should I have?" he replied. Skip was not the sharpest rock, but he was beginning to read something into Ashley's words. Skip asked Ashley why a woman would be calling him. Ashley's response was matter-of-fact. She said that the woman would be telling Skip that her husband was having an affair with Ashley. Skip, the blind soul that he was, asked Ashley why that would be. Suddenly, as Ashley began to speak, it hit Skip like a ton of bricks. Ashley's mouth was moving a mile a minute, as it usually did when she was nervous. Skip was picking up bits and pieces, but the picture was slowly coming together.

Skip finally said, "But the story the woman was to tell me isn't true, is it?"

Ashley responded with a disposed smile, and said, "Well, it might be."

The tether was back and Skip crashed hard. He saw himself on the floor crying in disbelief. Surely there is some mistake, he thought, but Ashley just kept talking and apologizing. Could this really be happening? How many times would Skip ask himself this question, "Did she really cheat on me while I was going through cancer rehabilitation?" and "Could it get any lower for either of them than this?"

Wow! Lots of questions with no answers. Skip had heard enough. Ashley kept talking, saying that it was the other guy who pursued her, and that she didn't want any part of it. This was the initial "big lie" that calmed Skip down for a moment as he tried to regain his composure.

"Who is this bastard?"

"Someone from work that you don't know," she said. "He was my supervisor and coerced me into this situation."

Now Skip didn't know what to believe. His grief cycle had just turned the corner to anger as Ashley told him this news. She kept speaking the same party line and Skip kept listening. Skip was not the violent type, so there was not even a thought of getting the gun or physically harming Ashley. He was, however, buying into her story about this bastard being the bad guy. Still, something smelled wrong. Skip and Ashley lived next to Margaret and her husband Daniel, who was a brilliant attorney. Skip made Ashley go over there right then and ask Daniel if they had a case against this guy and the company for which Ashley worked. What was she going to do, say no? Ashley went next door and came back with information that was somewhat positive. If this guy was her supervisor and he used his position to garner sexual favors, this was clearly sexual harassment, among other things.

The bomb had dropped, and Skip was severely wounded. Ashley was taking on collateral damage. It was getting late. The shells just kept hitting him, each one echoing a different form that someone had slept with his wife. No matter the circumstances, guilty or innocent, the event happened and must be handled. Skip's usual semi-psychotic way of dealing with issues was to bury them in the deepest, darkest, most remote part of his mind. The cancer was one thing. This was another. While the cancer could be killing him from the inside, the affair was killing him from the outside. Neither would ever go away, and both would be harshly tied together forever—at least forever on this earth.

†

Skip should have contacted a counselor immediately, but he was still stung from the news. He thought he needed to hear more details from Ashley. In hindsight, he should have left this one alone. Ashley told Skip that the furtive adultery lasted about six months, with about the same number of encounters. The sex took place mostly in hotels, but also in their

Toyota Camry. Skip stopped her there and said, "I want that car sold by the weekend." Ashley nodded politely. Skip grilled Ashley, but he had heard enough. He was also thinking that it was more mutual than she led him to believe. Maybe it was the part when she mentioned that they had begun a relationship that gave Skip this idea.

✝

Skip confided in those closest to him and shared the story of the infidelity. He got David Gorham on the phone and talked things out. David always had a way of putting things in perspective and casting a positive light on difficult circumstances. Skip couldn't remember David's advice after hanging up; he just remembered the teary emotions stirred up by their conversation. He would have more talks with David in the days to come. Skip's friend Steve Ferguson came by and Skip told him the news. Steve was a devout Christian and prayed with Skip. They put the whole issue into God's hands, which is where it should be. Skip knew that God would give him as much as he could take, and no more. Skip wanted and needed to believe this scripture, for Skip was sinking and was barely holding his head above water. Steve had suggested talking to some of the pastors at the church and seeking Christian counseling. It was too early for Skip to think about the counseling but, in hindsight, it should have been near the top of his to-do list. One of the pastors and a good friend of Skip's, Roy Harris, paid a visit after receiving a phone call from Steve Ferguson. Roy was the most pleasant and optimistic person he had ever met. He came over to the house and sat with Skip for a while. Skip was still very emotional, so he broke down in tears with just about everybody that came to see him. How could God possibly use a frail and weak man such as this to carry out any work in the name of the Kingdom? From Moses to Jesus and a plethora of men and women in between, God picked the least likely to perform a task most unsuited to them, but this hadn't occurred to Skip just yet. Not even close. Skip was in deep and just trying to climb out of the hole. The subject never came up, but if someone were to ask Skip if he would be of help to anyone, he most certainly would have said no.

Skip waited with Roy Harris in Greg Wood's office for Greg to arrive. Greg was a busy man running a mega church but took the time to visit with one of his flock, which Skip truly appreciated. Skip had been involved in the orphanage sponsored by West Cooper and several other projects, so he knew Greg on a first-name basis. It didn't hurt that Roy had made the call to set up the meeting. Greg first passed on his sympathies and said that although he had never gone through something like that, he knew that Skip was suffering dearly. After the initial small talk, which really wasn't small at all, Greg presented options to Skip based upon the Scriptures. He told Skip that he basically had two choices. The first was that he had the right to leave and divorce Ashley as a result of her adulterous affair. This, biblically, was grounds for divorce. Skip was wondering if they could stone her as well, but Greg never mentioned that Old Testament tradition. The second choice was to forgive her and stay together and attempt to reconcile their differences. Skip would actually need to forgive Ashley and Bob under both scenarios, as God forgives us as we sin against him. Skip thanked both Roy and Greg for taking the time to counsel him. He would consider their words very carefully.

Skip had a young family, and he was raised in the Catholic Church where divorce was frowned upon. And Ashley wanted to be forgiven and believed that she had been forgiven by God. She wanted the family to stay together and try to make things right. So, it was settled; they would remain married and attempt to work things out.

Ashley and Bob seemed to simultaneously drift apart, as the word had spread to their spouses. The sex, lies, and forbidden behavior was behind them, and they each moved on in their own way, with the mutual hope of reconciling their current spousal relationships. Easier said than done; the trust and bonds had been broken and battered. God could perform miracles, and Skip could think of one or two that might make his life on this earth a little easier.

Chapter 14

MAKING THE ROUNDS

†

Skip was on the mend and now going out of the house for his physical therapy. He walked gingerly still, and his arm remained in a sling most of the time. When he went to the physical therapist for the first time on site, they couldn't believe what terrible shape he was in. The first thing they did was try to build up his strength with a combination of walking in a pool against a resistant current and walking on a treadmill. These were formidable tasks in the early phases. The one thing that hadn't been mentioned to Skip was the buoyancy of his arm under the water. Out of the water, Skip could not move his arm an inch in an upward position. However, underwater, he was able to bring his arm up and down with the resistance being good for the atrophic muscles. The physical therapy consisted of these exercises for several weeks, as Skip had still not regained any strength in his legs or his upper body.

✝

The mission trip to Ecuador was still months away, and Skip was hoping that he would still be able to make it, along with Caroline, who was now in the eighth grade. It was a small contingent made up of two or three grown-ups and about a dozen middle school and high school-age kids. The mission was called Project Happy Feet, as they were to bring shoes to children in Quito, Ecuador. The cost was about $1500 per person, and Skip was concerned about the money with his mounting medical bills and lack of income. If it was God's plan for him and Caroline to go, then it would happen; that was the way Skip looked at it. They were all about collecting shoes and raising money. Skip and Caroline created a fundraising letter and mailed it to every friend and relative that they knew. It was quite successful, raising almost enough money for one of their trips. West Cooper had a shoe collection day one Sunday where members of the congregation could bring in new or gently worn shoes to be taken on the mission trip to Ecuador. Shoes were brought by the hundreds. Between West Cooper and donations from local stores, there seemed to be as many shoes as the group could carry to Ecuador in their duffle bags. Skip had about four to five months to get himself together for the trip.

✝

Gradually his legs regained strength. The small pool with the resistant water flow was the perfect rehabilitation tool that Skip needed. Because Skip was in such bad shape, the physical therapists hadn't even begun to work on the arm yet. When it was time to continue with the arm rehab, the exercises were very basic and mundane. Skip would place his arm on a table and try to use his hand and fingers to stretch out his arm as far as he could. He also did this standing up against a wall. He would use his left arm to place his right arm on the wall. Then, he had to use his hand and fingers to get his arm to climb the wall. This was a very difficult task at first, and it never got any easier. He eventually moved on to more profound objects like balls and weight equipment, but he was seriously injured and they knew he would recover only a small percentage of his overall functioning.

✝

He was still too close to the cancer and the chemo to go back to visit 5 South at Roper Hospital—too many memories and most of them bad. So, he decided to volunteer at the State Medical University just down the road. This would take his mind off his own circumstances while getting the chance, he hoped, to work with others. Becoming a volunteer at the State Medical University was about as easy to do as getting in to its medical school. Form after picture after another form. Skip wondered why all the security just to do a little volunteering. After making it through the gauntlet of obstacles, several weeks later he was officially issued a University Volunteer identification card. Skip volunteered on Sunday evenings, when he thought family would probably have left for the weekend and the floor would have few visitors. With BA and MBA in hand, Skip was now in charge, somewhat, of pushing the snack cart around to each room on the cancer floor. He would come in a little before his six o'clock evening shift to organize everything and see what was in the fridge and cabinets. Skip rarely, if ever, saw a doctor on the floor at this time of day, but there was a plethora of nurses scurrying around, both male and female. With snack cart loaded, Skip began his volunteer venture down the hall to Room 212. Even though he knew what to expect, he was still rather shy and had butterflies in his stomach when he knocked on the door.

✝

Skip's rehabilitation was improving and so was his optimism about the Ecuador mission trip. Money had been raised for Caroline, and Skip was praying about the remainder. The trip was now only several weeks away, so plans were being finalized. What money had been collected from the participants thus far was given to the church, which made up the short fall to purchase the airline tickets. The flight would go from Charleston to Atlanta, and then to Houston and on to Quito. The mission group met at least once and often twice a week in the time closest to departure. They all had the same duffle bags and used them to hold the myriad of shoes that were collected. There was room for just about everything collected, which made the group happy. The team had identical shirts and crosses made up to wear, establishing their identities as they would roll around the world. Tickets were in hand, and bags were packed with shoes. It was just a waiting game now until the flight was scheduled to leave.

✝

The door to Room 212 was slightly ajar as Skip poked his head around the door to take a look inside. He saw an elderly white woman, probably in her early eighties lying in bed dozing off. Skip wasn't sure whether to go in with the snack cart and disturb her. Since this was his first room, he decided to go in. The woman was momentarily startled but told Skip to come in, in a hushed tone. Skip opened the door just wide enough to bring the cart in so as not to disturb the woman any more than he already had. Skip told her that he was a volunteer and pushed the snack cart around to each room and was wondering if she wanted something. She didn't want anything from the cart, but she needed a glass of water with ice. Her ice bucket was empty, so Skip went to the ice machine to fill the bucket for her and poured her a fresh glass of water. Skip asked if she would like him to turn the television on or do anything else. She just wanted to talk. Skip assumed, as when he was having his chemotherapy treatments, that there were always family members visiting patients, checking up on them, and advocating for their needs. This woman had no one. She was a widow of many years and had two children who lived on the West Coast. So Skip mostly listened. The woman talked about her deceased husband, her kids and grandkids, and everything in between. Skip looked at his watch and started to get nervous. He had the entire floor to visit and had spent over half an hour talking to her. Skip kindly excused himself and said he needed to visit others down the hall. She grabbed his hand and gave him a big smile. On his way out, Skip ran into one of the male nurses in the hall who asked, "Were you just in with Mrs. Jennings?" Skip said that he was. The nurse told Skip that Mrs. Jennings wasn't supposed to make it much longer, as she had stage IV breast cancer. The nurse continued his rounds, but this stopped Skip dead in his tracks. The reality of cancer had hit him again, and he wasn't sure if he could handle it. What would Jesus do?

†

The group huddled together outside of the USAir terminal and said a final prayer before boarding their flight for Ecuador. All were present and accounted for and ready to go. One of Caroline's friends, Jesse, was very sick the day of the flight and wasn't sure that she could make it. They all prayed for her healing, and somehow she made it on the plane and began a slow recovery from whatever was ailing her. The large group of adults and kids would get stares during their journey. There would have been one day, not too many years ago, in which Skip might not even have glanced their way or given them a second thought. Now, God had got him going out into the world singing the praises of Jesus. It was rumored that Quito, Ecuador, had one of the top ten worst runways in the world. Apparently, it was situated between two mountain ranges at ten thousand feet above sea level on the equator. What could one do? Just hang on and enjoy the ride, Skip supposed. Quito is a little west of Charleston in the big picture and an hour behind on the clock. There wouldn't be any jet lag, just flight lag from a long time being in the air.

The trip was organized by West Cooper but was the brainchild of Seve and Michelle Harmon. They were the feet on the ground in Ecuador, and the group would be staying with them. Both were fluent in Spanish, as was one of the adults in our group. Seve and Michelle were married and used their home to support mission trips from all over the world. Skip's group would be the first Happy Feet group from West Cooper. Seve met Greg Wood on a trip back to the states, and the benevolent relationship had begun. After clearing customs, which wasn't as difficult as they had anticipated, a bus and driver met them outside the airport for the ride back to the Harmons'. It was late, the middle of the night, so most slept during the journey through the Ecuadorian countryside. It was the beginning, the alpha of their journey, and so the group arrived with some trepidation.

✝

Skip left a slight crack in Mrs. Jennings' door as he left to find his next room. The corridor was T-shaped with rooms on each side of the hall. Skip wondered how he would take care of all of these patients. He was the only volunteer that he knew of thus far on Sunday evenings. Skip was surprised to see two armed guards in the next room he entered. There was a young black man lying in the bed with the traditional bags of chemotherapy hanging bedside. The guards never spoke to the young man or Skip while he was in the room. Skip asked him if he could get him anything, and he said, "Yeah, can you get me out of here?" Skip had sandwiches on the cart, and he asked for the turkey sandwich and a coke. Skip gladly gave him the food and was rather quick to leave, not attempting to strike up a conversation. Skip said good-bye and left the room. He could only assume that he was serving time at some jail or prison, and they were letting him out to get his chemotherapy. He didn't know what he had done, but he was being paid back in spades with his suffering. Skip had the luxury of going home to a beautiful house and loving family and friends. This man was going back to jail, where he was sure he wasn't given the golden glove treatment. Skip shook off the sadness and regrouped before entering the next room. Inside he saw a very young black girl, who could have been no more than thirteen or fourteen. Skip asked her what kind of cancer she had, and she told him that she was suffering from sickle-cell anemia. Skip wondered what she was doing on this floor, but he would later learn of other patients on the cancer ward that suffered from sickle cell. They took a similar pharmaceutical protocol to that of cancer patients, which is why they were intermingled. God took no mercy on the race of the patient, as there appeared to be almost an equal number of black and white patients. Skip gave the little girl a soda and some crackers and was on his way.

Skip followed the same routine each Sunday night. He was slowly getting into the swing of it and now knew most of the nursing staff and the occasional doctor or two. He would load his cart with whatever was available and make his rounds. The patients, with few exceptions, were generally different week to week. Some stayed longer after surgery and some shorter due to the length of their chemo protocol.

On one occasion, Skip entered a room with a woman about his age in the bed with who appeared to be her husband beside her. Skip could tell she had been crying and wasn't sure what to do. Skip had been volunteering for over a month now but was reticent about saying anything about God or praying for anyone. Skip introduced himself and, as he usually did, he asked the woman what type of cancer she had. She told him it was ovarian, and that she wasn't doing well. Skip almost always told the patients that he had cancer and was a cancer survivor to this point. He felt it brought a bond between him and the patients, and it almost always did. Skip would often retell the story that he just wanted to see someone who had gone through this hell come out on the other side. His cancer was so rare that he never met anyone who had Ewing's sarcoma or the similar bone cancer known as osteosarcoma. Skip elaborated a little more on his trials and tribulations with cancer over the past few years, and he mentioned how God gave him strength when he was losing hope. Skip immediately noticed a gleam in her eyes as he mentioned God and hope. Skip would tell her what he had come to tell all the patients that he conversed with: "We are only here on this earth for a short period of time, and I hope and pray that God heals you to live another day. More importantly, make sure you know where your heart is and that it belongs to Jesus, because eternity is forever, and life without Jesus is eternity without hope." This would come to be Skip's mantra with those who were receptive. In a place where no human wants to be, lonely and without hope, almost everyone that Skip encountered would listen to him to some degree. He wasn't really proselytizing, but it came from his heart, and he felt that those in this place needed to hear it. It would be interesting to know how many people who came to the cancer floor were believers and held some belief in God, because Skip found that almost without exception, every patient that he serviced was interested in hearing about his cancer journey and the part that God played in it. It could be as brief as saying a quick prayer for someone, to sitting down and telling them about Benny Hinn and other miraculous events that happened throughout his saga. Skip was helping to bring hope to an otherwise hopeless place.

✝

The first thing they did when they got to Seve and Michelle's residence was crash. It was still the middle of the night, so sleep for a few more hours was on the minds of most. The coolness crept into the bunkhouse where the men and boys were residing. The sun made its way up across the beautiful Ecuadorian sky and woke the group. Skip was surprised by the dichotomy between what appeared to be a tropical climate, complete with fruit trees that you might see in Florida, and the morning chill that was in the air. Because Quito sits some ten thousand feet above sea level on the equator, it brings with it a temperate zone unlike many others. The temperature fluctuated in a tight range around seventy degrees Fahrenheit, and without the humidity the group was accustomed to in the Lowcountry. Seve and Michelle had breakfast going and, in the land of the coffee bean, they drank freeze-dried coffee with their breakfast. Seve was one heck of a cook and laid out a spread of everything from eggs to sausage and all the in-betweens. There wasn't a lot of down time at base camp, as Seve had each day mapped out with a full itinerary. The kids ventured outside and glimpsed the house and the neighborhood. Probably the most striking feature of each house was not that it had a fence, but that the fence was laden with broken glass at the top, which served as barbed wire, it seemed. Seve assured the group that the neighborhood was safe; it was just the way things were done in this part of town. The geography of the neighborhood was such that it was partially flat and partially embanked on a huge cliff. What surprised the kids was that there were no goats, but cows grazing on the very steep terrain. The house seemed more like a compound than a home but was a wonderful spot to use as a springboard for the mission.

After breakfast, a bus pulled up to take the group on its first mission. One thing Skip had to say was that Seve made it much easier to get around Ecuador than it was for he and Ashley to backpack across Europe. Seve had organized the week so that what they first saw of the town would be less striking or intrusive to them and would work its way up—or rather down—as the week went on.

✝

Skip thought it was strange that there was rarely a nurse or doctor in any of the rooms that he would visit. It really shouldn't have surprised him though, as it was the same when he was at 5 South over at Roper Hospital. Not to say that the nurses were not doing their jobs; it just seemed a little odd that the rooms were always empty with the exception of the patient and Skip.

Skip met another young man about his age watching television in one of the rooms. He had a baseball game on, so Skip struck up a conversation about the Braves and how well they were looking this year. Skip told him that when he himself was doing chemo in the spring, he longed to get to Turner Field with the family to take in a game. Skip made the man laugh when he told him that he used to watch the games at Roper with an older gentleman who would drink beer during the games. Skip had always meant to ask Dr. Barker if he really wrote the prescription for the beer, or was his wife, with the aid of a nurse, bringing it in for him. Either way, it was priceless. As it typically did, the conversation led to cancer and what type of cancer the patient had. He was stricken with a form of brain cancer called astrocytoma, grade three. This had a poor prognosis, so Skip went to work on his mission of hope. Skip wasn't sure if he was a God-fearing man before getting the brain cancer, but after a long talk with Skip about this just being a short-term temporal existence, his fears seemed to subside and a peace came over him. Skip knew that he was at the right place at the right time performing the work that God wanted him to do: to give hope to the hopeless and strength to the weary.

✝

Day one had the group visiting a church on the outskirts of Quito. The pastor was a friend of Seve's and decided this would be a great place for the group to start its evangelicalism. The initial bus ride gave them their first view of the Quito region. The countryside leading into the city was breathtaking and beautiful. The mountain streams and steep cliffs gave way to a slightly flatter terrain as they approached the city. Small neighborhood streets were lined with petite shops and food stores that gave the area a real local flair. Not a McDonald's or Burger King to be found. Everyone was amazed at the jagged glass-top fences, which seemed to be ubiquitous whether in the countryside or the city. The ride from Seve's compound to the church was approximately an hour, but time went by quickly as they took in sights they had never seen before. Several of the teens had their iPods playing to the dismay of the adults. Teens would be teens. They had to have their music.

The church looked exuberant under the bright sun as the bus pulled out back to park. It was a Sunday, so the church was having its regular service, and the group was its guests. Almost the entire contemporary service was in Spanish, but it didn't seem to affect the group, for the melodies were enchanting and, for the most part, the same hymns sung at West Cooper. There were approximately fifty people in the small congregational area, and everyone had a wide smile as they sang. Hands were even waved in the air. The praise and worship lasted for about half an hour, and then the group broke for lunch. The pastor had provided food for his congregation as well as for the missionaries. The young children sat in one room off to the side, and the adults sat in another room. There were several Ecuadorian women and a few of the teenage girls looking out for and playing with the young ones as they ate.

The pastor spoke English and told the group a little bit about his flock. Most were not working due to the economy, and this would probably be the only meal that they would receive that day. Most had nothing more than the shirts on their backs, but they still had happiness and peace about them. How different from the American population that seemed to never have enough. Less is more is the pervasive attitude of the believers here, knowing that God would take care of their earthly needs. Skip had been preaching the less is more motto for some time now, although it was an entirely different scenario over here.

While the men were talking, the women were cleaning, and the mission kids were coloring and making beads with the Ecuadorian children. There was an instant bond between the Happy Feet group and the local congregation. But this would not be one of the places where the group would hand out shoes. Those would be saved for later in the week.

✝

Ashley was either unimpressed or unfazed by Skip's Sunday night visits to the hospital. Caroline would ask where he was going, and he would say to the hospital to help people with cancer. Ashley was always so busy, so Skip usually just swung by the local Taco Bell for a few fifty-nine cent tacos for dinner on his way downtown. Skip had the routine down by heart at the hospital. He would greet whoever was around, load his cart, and then begin his rounds. Then, he noticed a change. Skip had been volunteering on Sunday nights for almost three months now, but it was getting harder and harder for him to make the journey each week. Skip was still less than a year removed from his own chemotherapy nightmare and was still dealing seriously with the arm issues. It was wearing him down. He would get teary eyed with patients, and sometimes he would cry with them. This emotional toll had its benefits, but Skip was still too close to it; it still hit home too hard.

Skip's predicament was that he felt it was his calling to give back to those who needed to hear his story of survival and success as well as to hear the Word of God. Maybe he was still too close to his own situation to delve into the lives of other sufferers. Not everyone is a cancer hero. Most aren't. Celebrities like Lance Armstrong donated time and effort to the cause, but that was another world and another game entirely. Many run in the Susan G. Komen fight against breast cancer. Many don't. Each cancer survivor is unique. Skip wanted to do more, but he just couldn't. After all, he wasn't really out of the woods yet, and he still worried that things could change at any moment. Every cancer survivor would like to encourage or pass on a message of hope to others but, just like Skip, they had their own fears; and many are simply sucked back into the vacuous world again as if the cancer had never happened. Ultimately, it is God's will. Only He knows why we are here, and what we are meant to do.

✝

Skip and Ashley's relationship had changed little since the affair. Ashley was apologetic, as one might expect, and thought they should get involved in counseling to get things right again. Skip was not a big counseling fan. Everyone he ever knew who was in the profession was crazier than he was. Needless to say, counseling never got off the ground. Skip still held on to too much anger and grief to allow anyone else to enter his life to try to fix it. Skip made Ashley's life a living hell for the longest time with his passive-aggressive tactics and coldness. This was the course he had set for himself in the short term; he would follow it to see where it might lead.

✝

It was just past Christmas, wintertime in Ecuador. The trip started the day after Christmas, and the group would return home the day before public schools started again. This meant they would celebrate New Year's Eve in Quito, along with the Ecuadorians. A unique local custom was to burn the mask or mannequin figure of a celebrity or politician in effigy. Skip and the adults traveled to a part of Quito with Seve to find something they could use this New Year's night. They stumbled across many but ended up with a mannequin of Hillary Clinton, who may or may not have been running for president or some other political office at the time. In addition to the mannequin, a sufficient amount of fireworks were procured for the night's festivities. All went off without a hitch. After dinner, the mannequin was set up and traditionally burned at sunset, and the fireworks were ablaze.

To prepare for their first Happy Feet mission in the morning, they performed the ceremony on each other that night before bed. Prayer, cleansing of the feet, and putting on shoes was done by one to another. It was a peaceful time, but everyone was wondering what would happen the next day.

The bus rolled in early as usual, and the group loaded up. The buses were meant to hold at least fifty passengers, but barely half the seats were filled. Seve led the group to another church in another part of Quito. As they got closer, they realized they were not in Kansas anymore. The roads were rougher, and they noticed more people about. The last several miles were a combination of dirt and asphalt, making for a rocky ride. The bus pulled up to what looked like an empty church, but as soon as the gates opened they were greeted by the warm smile of the church pastor and his wife. Several other Ecuadorian staff members were there to help them set up the makeshift shoe store. Everyone had a job to do, and it was all avant-garde. Music was arranged for background noise, and shoes were organized by size and type. This was all done before the parishioners arrived. Everyone was a little nervous. Bowls and towels were placed before the dozen or so folding chairs that were set up. They were ready. Skip would remember this day for the rest of his life.

The pastor and his wife spoke with Seve and were introduced to the group. They had nothing. Skip felt so sad; he pulled out a twenty dollar bill and gave it to the pastor and mumbled some words about trying to help out. The pastor was grateful and spoke back in broken English. One moment of silence, and the next a small army had gathered outside the church. Apparently the word of the shoe handout had gotten around the neighborhood, if one could call it that, and people were waiting patiently to come inside. Seve and the pastor were very strict with the rules, so only the families of children who attended the church would get the shoes because they wanted to make it special for the congregation. It was obvious that those who showed up had little to nothing in the way of clothing or money. Those who could find work made on average ten dollars a day.

It was one of the most remarkable events that Skip had ever witnessed. As the crowd filtered in slowly, each person took his or her place at a chair. Mostly mothers with their children were looking for shoes for their children's otherwise bare feet.

Skip's first assignment was to wash the feet of those who sat, as Jesus did to the apostles during the last supper. He had a bowl of clean, warm water and soap and cleansed and dried each foot. One of the other missionaries would then place the shoes on the child. There were also adults and the elderly who visited in need of shoes as well. The low, contemporary music playing in the background made for a perfect setting. One of the kids had set up a printer and camera so the group could take and give a picture of the person with their new pair of shoes. Skip was emotional. The things we take for granted at home are gold to those in other lands. The lines seemed endless, but there was no chaos.

Skip had been working on the feet of a young teenage girl. One of the missionaries, a teenage girl herself, remarked to Skip that they were all out of the young girl's shoe size. They told her this several times before she understood and, her head hanging low, she headed for the door. In a flash, the teenage missionary took her tennis shoes off her own feet and put them on the feet of the Ecuadorian teen. What an act of kindness, thought Skip. God truly touched this young American's heart. They all hugged afterwards and sent her on her way, with a smile on her face.

A scuffle was taking place outside the church. Skip overheard some conversation and went to take a look for himself. By this time, most of the congregation had come through and received their blessings. However, on the outside, as far as one could see, mothers with children were waiting for shoes for their children. The look in the eyes of the mothers who were sent away empty-handed left an indelible mark on Skip. All they wanted was shoes, and the group could not deliver. The pastor tried to calm the crowd, and slowly they trickled away. Like the fish and the loaves of bread that Jesus had multiplied for the masses, Skip wished they could do the same with the shoes. Why didn't Skip think that God would give him the power to do this? Could it have been his lack of belief that it could happen? Why didn't he hold up his own pair of shoes and ask God to multiply them? Skip had no answers. What was in reality a marvelous day of healing and helping ended bittersweet. God bless those people.

To their surprise and disappointment, Skip told the head nurse at the hospital that next week would be his last for a while. She said they would be sorry to see him go, as it was nice to have an extra set of hands around, albeit untrained hands. Skip decided that he would deliver his mantra of healing and prayer to all those willing to partake this particular evening. As with most nights, just about everyone was receptive to his prayers. When visiting twenty or thirty rooms and all but a few are willing to listen, the success rate is pretty high. Keep in mind that like 5 South at Roper Hospital, this was usually the last stop for most on this earth. Skip would run into a full gamut, from adamant believers to those who had never really heard the Word. Without exception, everyone wanted to know that there was a better place than where they were currently, and if Skip could help them see it, all the better. Most thanked Skip for the insight and for visiting. People were really surprised when they learned he was a cancer survivor. At this point, with hair grown back and weight gain beginning, he did not look like a cancer patient. When his arm was not in its sling, Skip would tell the patients about the surgery and the prosthesis, which they generally marveled at. Some would even offer to help Skip serve them the beverage or snack. But Skip assured them he was fine and continued on. He served his last patient and cleaned up his cart and put away the leftover food. Skip ran into the hospital chaplain on his way out, and they exchanged words. Skip told him that he would be leaving next Sunday, as he needed a respite from the volunteer work. The chaplain asked Skip if he wanted to talk about it, and Skip just mentioned that he was still too close to the cancer and the situation, and he needed a break from seeing all the suffering and pain. The chaplain understood totally and prayed a quick healing prayer for Skip before he went on his way. On the drive home, Skip would always reflect on the evening but was usually glad that it was over. The dichotomy of helping those in need and helping himself was resolved in his favor for now.

†

Their bags were packed in preparation for an early wake-up call the following morning. The group was to leave Seve and Michelle's house by four in the morning to catch a six o'clock plane. They were on schedule as far as the missionary group went. However, once they had boarded the plane, a dense fog began to roll in and grounded the flight for several hours. Most of the adults slept while the teens listened to music and dozed in and out of consciousness. Once the fog had finally cleared, the captain gave the go-ahead for takeoff. Due to the plane's idling for so long, the captain told the passengers that they would be stopping briefly in Panama to refuel before heading back to Houston. They were probably on the tarmac in Panama for an hour or so before heading off again. Another country the kids could say they visited upon returning home. With everything being pushed back because of the fog in Quito, they missed their scheduled flight from Houston to Atlanta. This would mean spending the night in Houston, and the kids would miss the first day of school after winter break. They were heartbroken as one can imagine. The return to Charleston was essentially uneventful from that point forward. All said their good-byes and hugged and kissed as they each went their own separate way.

Skip knew that his life had forever changed. Ecuador was a place of both beauty and utter poverty. Such images, both good and bad, were burnt in his mind forever. His hope was that this trip would also show Caroline and the other kids that there was a big world out there and not everyone was living like they were in Charleston. While this hit home with them for a while, they slowly got sucked back into the upper middle class of the Charlestonian lifestyle. However, Skip believed that deep down in their hearts, they had been changed for the better, and a part of Ecuador would remain inside of them to keep their lives in balance.

✝

It was his last Sunday, so Skip got ready to head downtown to the hospital. Ashley had cooked a Sunday dinner that afternoon, so Skip wasn't particularly hungry when he left. Her demeanor toward Skip was still cold, but who could blame her? Skip's reaction to the affair was beyond reproach.

Or was it? He said good-bye and headed out one last time. Skip had seen life and he had seen death on his journeys through cancer wards. Death was a natural part of life. What concerned Skip, though, was what happened after death. Skip was a true believer that knowing God and believing in Jesus was the right ticket to punch for all the right reasons. On his last night, he steadfastly passed this message to those who were willing to listen. Everyone, with the exception of several who were sleeping, did listen. People in situations like these want to know the answers to these questions. Skip didn't have all the answers—that's for sure. He didn't know if he had any of the answers. Skip had come to realize that people are going to do what they want to do, whether it's right or wrong or in-between. However, when it came to life after death, attitudes changed and people did become more interested in what others had to say. Skip spoke his mind on his last night at the hospital, and people liked what he had to say.

Chapter 15
WHAT REALLY MATTERS

†

The game of life had led Skip down a path he couldn't have imagined in a hundred years. Everyone has their trials and tribulations, but when it hits close to home, it especially tingles. Things never were really the same again between Skip and Ashley. A bond had been broken and trust had been compromised. The give and take from each always seemed to take place at different times, resulting in maintaining a status quo of grief and regret. This intolerable situation went on for years. Neither Ashley nor Skip liked the state of affairs, but Skip was comfortable with staying the course. His passive aggressiveness was his outlet. He was determined to keep the family together for the sake of the children, regardless of his ill feelings toward Ashley.

†

Unhealthy would be a good word to describe the current situation at the Sibley household, as well as Skip's state of mind. From the children's standpoint, there was no difference in the relationship between Mom and Dad. They were still too young, although Caroline was now a young teenager who probably knew more than she let on. Foster, on the other hand, had no thoughts of impending doom as it related to the relationship between his parents, for he was too young.

Skip was quiet and becoming more reclusive as time passed. He rarely spoke to Ashley but would listen to her talk about this and that. Most discussions centered on finances, or the lack of them. They had built up so much equity in the house for the longest time that money was never really an issue. However, the real estate market in Charleston and most of the country was beginning to decline, and with it, the feeling of disposable income was declining. Skip seemed to ignore not only their financial issues, but just about everything else as well. Although his faith was still strong, he didn't attend church on a regular basis. Although he had a great many friends, he began to withdraw from social settings. Things were not good in the mind of Skip Sibley. On one hand, he wanted to click his heals together and make everything go back to the way it was before the cancer. On the other, cancer opened his eyes to a world that he had never known. He only now understood why it was said by some that cancer can be the best thing that can happen to you, live or die. He knew this well but had difficulty processing it all. He appreciated the sound of birds singing and children laughing and could slow down at times and take in the smell of the salt air of the ocean. But he was fighting too many demons to take full advantage of his gift of remission. He was and always would be thankful for the gift of eternal life that came with his rebirth in Christ as a result of his illness. This alone was worth the price of admission as a cancer survivor. Skip had to learn how to die before he could learn how to live.

✝

It was only a matter of time before Ashley and Skip would separate. Counseling had been attempted intermittently. It was mostly the unwillingness of Skip to forgive Ashley for what she had done to him and the family. Throw in a life-changing cancer, and you have a recipe for disaster. Skip was unreceptive to the attempts at reconciliation. He just couldn't get past things. He felt wounded and betrayed and was stuck in a bad place mentally. He knew he was supposed to forgive sin as God forgives his sins. That was easier said than done. Skip's mind was not in the cycle of forgiveness, and he languished in anger and self-pity.

Ashley had been hinting around that she had had enough and was going to leave. Skip ignored the warning signs and continued his lurid denial. It shouldn't have, but it caught Skip by surprise. One morning he awoke in a cold sweat to find Ashley and Caroline gone. Skip ran frantically to Foster's room but saw that he was still asleep in his own bed. A cryptic note was left with a brief explanation. Life, again, would never be the same.

✝

Ashley had rented a house across town and had a room for Caroline and Foster in it. Caroline spent the majority of her time with Ashley in the new rental property, and Foster spent most of his time in Bay Club with Skip. The innuendos were coming back to Skip. Ashley had asked him on occasion if he wouldn't be happier or more comfortable somewhere other than the Bay Club house. Skip ignored her as usual and finally pushed her to the breaking point. If he didn't need therapy before, he certainly needed it now. The thought never occurred to Skip, or most like him, that he might have a problem with depression. It had been over five years since the cancer, surgery, and the affair. Skip was detaching slowly from the world without even realizing it. He was still on the disability, so he had no interaction on a professional or social basis with anyone really. As much as they both were tormented, Skip never thought that Ashley might leave him one day. He assumed life would continue on and maybe get better, or maybe not. He was content to have the family together under one roof. When this change of events occurred, it once again sent him, without realizing it, into new depths of despair. Skip made attempts to talk Ashley out of leaving and returning to the Bay Club house, but she would have none of it. At this point, she had pretty much removed herself from attending church on a regular basis and was probably getting advice from her friends, many of whom were divorced themselves. Ashley would not give the traditional family another go. She was determined to leave Skip and to try to maintain life with the children as normal as possible. As detached as Skip had been, he had started to get it when Ashley moved out. He was ready for counseling, but Ashley was beyond reconciliation. Skip thought of the children. He wondered if Ashley thought of the children and what it would do to them psychologically. He always thought that she put herself first, being an only child. Skip recounted the days when the kids were young when she would feed herself breakfast first, and then see what the kids wanted to eat. She blamed it on low blood sugar or some other bull.

It all went back to the first time Ashley was left to care for Caroline after her mother left. Ashley was like a deer in the headlights, without a clue of what to do. Believe it or not, Skip seemed to have the more maternal instinct with Caroline and Foster than Ashley. Skip felt that Ashley would always take care of herself and her needs first, whereas Skip always looked out for the kids as his top priority.

Faith. You can't see it, touch it, or smell it. You just have to believe. Skip's faith was being seriously tested, but he never once wavered. His cancer and life from it had given him faith that he hoped would carry him through the rest of his days on Earth. God was good to Skip. God could have taken him to be with him many times throughout his young life: the car accident in high school, the cancer, and any number of other accidents that came his way. But God didn't. Skip wore his faith on his sleeve like a badge of courage. He was not the over-the-top evangelical, but if you wanted to talk about faith, he would listen and tell you his story. If he had it to do all over again, he would be a theologian or a monk and spend his time on what is really important in this world: preparing you for the next.

✝

Ashley made the transition from family under one roof to family divided as seamlessly as possible. She moved several times during the separation, all very quietly to avoid confusing or upsetting the children. Skip maintained residence in the Bay Club house, but it was not nearly the same. The one thing about being separated or divorced with kids is that one usually has to interact with one's estranged spouse. For Skip, this was a daily nightmare. At first, Skip could not bring himself to go to the place where Ashley was living. It was too hard. It hurt too badly. The problem was that he missed Caroline, and she didn't come back to the Bay Club house that often. Skip began making brief appearances, under the auspices of dropping off Foster, and actually entering the residence where Ashley was residing. It was painful. There was the same furniture, pictures (minus the ones with Skip), and some new things that sent Skip to the breaking point. He made a conscious effort to spend some time with Caroline and then leave as quickly as he could. Caroline, being a young teen, missed Skip, but also had her friends and a world of her own going on. Skip could vaguely understand it all. He wondered what Ashley had told Caroline about him that made her leave the Bay Club house. Caroline loved her daddy and wouldn't do anything to hurt him.

Skip had never mentioned anything about the affair to Caroline. She was old enough now to certainly understand if he did. Skip thought about it many times but decided against it. Several of those in his family and friendship circle were curious as to why he didn't tell Caroline. Ashley certainly wouldn't say anything bad about herself, would she? Skip likened telling Caroline about the affair to the belief in God or Jesus. People want proof that something happened. Moses in the Old Testament told the people of the one true God and brought them the commandments to live by. However, time and time again the Hebrews would wander, build idolatry, and fall from grace in not believing. Faith. As in the days of Moses, people knew in their hearts that there was a God, for Moses had received the Word to pass on to the Jews. People had changed very little in three thousand years. While they may suspect something, they may just as quickly forget it or not make it a part of their daily lives. This is one reason why God continued to make the Hebrews suffer. Knowing that there is an almighty omnipresent God, how could anyone deviate from his love? But the people did.

The same could be said in New Testament times with Jesus. The healings, the miracles, the linchpin of Christianity and the resurrection, were all witnessed by man and yet the people turned on Jesus in the end. How could this be? Jesus even raised the dead. Faith. The Son of God was put to death by his own people. He was virtually ignored in his hometown. Oh ye of little faith.

The same held true in Skip's mind about telling Caroline about the furtive affair. She would hear the story but would forget it shortly thereafter, and then how much better off would Skip have been? He wanted to tell her it wasn't his fault. He wanted to tell her about the affair, but he couldn't. He knew in time it wouldn't matter. Her young life would go on, and the affair could not be blamed on all future and past faults. This is why Skip held it close to the vest. Don't think it didn't widen the hole in his heart each day as he kept his mouth shut and went about his business. How many dark details can you tuck away in the cerebrum before it comes back to haunt you? How many times can you get knocked down before you say *no mas?*

Since Foster spent most of his time with Dad at the Bay Club house, Ashley would visit almost daily, usually in the evenings after work. Skip was amenable to this, since he basically had no choice. Ashley might stay for a few minutes or a few hours. It always felt like an eternity. Skip was still trying to persuade Ashley to come back but, as before, she said that they were just too different and that it would be better this way. She did not believe that Skip loved her anyway. Skip found it almost impossible at this time to show love and affection toward Ashley, since he was still holding onto the anger and grief of the affair. He wanted it to be like it was when they were in their twenties, prior to having children. He wanted to feel as he did in those days again but didn't know how to get there. How could she betray him by sleeping with another man? Would it have been different if Skip never found out? How badly did they talk about Skip? These and a myriad of other questions constantly circulated through Skip's mind, making him anxious and depressed, although he had no idea that his mental state was being altered.

The most horrific part for Skip would be when Ashley would leave each day. She would say good-bye to Foster, turn her back on Skip, and walk out the front door. It was like she was leaving Skip anew each day. It was like having a premonition each day of the door slamming shut on Skip's former life. Each day hurt as much as the first day. Skip wasn't sure whether Ashley was cognizant of what was going on or not, but it damaged Skip's psyche. This was not an occasional event; it went on for years. There were no more dark places for Skip's embattled issues to hide. His mind was dark and chaotic. He was not in a good place and didn't see any way out.

Chapter 16
REALITY SETS IN

✝

The riches were gone. The "For Sale" sign was up in front of the Bay Club house. Skip tried to postpone the sale as long as possible. Although far from perfect, he maintained a lifestyle, mental health aside, which kept him comfortable. Skip did not like change. When they bought the house, Skip remembered Ashley saying that it would be their "starter home" and that one day they would probably live on one of the islands surrounding Charleston. Skip managed to leverage each dollar very well from his younger days in the stock market. He had no idea it would end up like this. South Carolina. What was he doing there anyway? It was, after all, his idea to relocate closer to Ashley's family and farther away from DC and his troubled business relationships. Skip and the boys cashed in on their business at a decent time in the market. Anytime is probably pretty decent when you are handed almost a million dollars before you are thirty years old. They had just missed the beginning of the Internet bubble, though. If timing had been a little better and they had hung on for a little longer, who knows what the value of their little business might have been. They were a tad ahead of their time in becoming dot-com billionaires. Skip thought about that on occasion but wondered where that road would have led. Would he have spent his life surrounded by money and earthly pleasures? Would he have been brought down to that low rung on the totem pole that would bring him eternal life? It is hard to say. Was the cancer destined to come through genetics or other predetermined biological events, or did the stress and high-paced lifestyle push it over the edge?

Is there really "free will" in a biblical sense? Skip would often debate this with David Gorham and a few others who had an interest in this topic. In its most liberal sense, we are free to do what we like on Earth. We can walk, drop a glass, change jobs, or whatever the event might be. But is this free will? Skip used to think that it was, and he would argue just that. People have the ability to do what they want on this earth. Skip recalled the story of an atheist professor who would drop a pencil before class every day and then asked God not to let the pencil hit the ground. Day after day the pencil would hit the ground. Subtle tactics used by the liberal left in education to reeducate the youth of America. Skip bought into this and also said it was free will that let the pencil hit the ground each day. After all, the Old Testament days of miracles were behind us now, weren't they?

"But do we really have free will?" David Gorham would persist.

Let's start with heaven and hell. Don't those of us who are going to heaven have our names written in the Lamb's Book of Life?

"If this is so, how can there be free will?" David would ask.

Is there not predestination? Believers would say that God is, among other things, omniscient, omnipotent, and omnipresent. If God knew before we were even born that we were going to heaven or hell, how does that impact our free will? If you are in the Book, does it mean that you cannot be a satanic worshiper or Wiccan? If you had free will, surely you could make these choices. How could this be? Although not included in the Bible, the book of Revelation by Peter in the Gnostic books suggests something different. Peter has a conversation with Jesus whereby he asks how can an altruistic God sentence people to hell? Jesus responds, "I will let you in on a little secret; everyone will go to heaven." This book was excluded from the Bible for many reasons, but mostly because it might send the wrong message to believers, saying that you can do anything here on Earth, and God will welcome you with open arms in heaven. David and Skip would always discuss this and other topics in the Bible from Genesis to the end times.

✝

The time had finally come. It was moving day. The Bay Club house had sold for well below what it was worth several years prior, but Skip and Ashley still managed to pull a decent amount of equity out of the property. "It would have been a lot more," muttered Skip, "if it didn't have to be split in half." Ashley relocated to a larger house in a nicer part of town with larger rooms for the kids, especially Caroline. The rental also came with a hefty price tag. This must have been somewhat disconcerting to Ashley since she really had no income; her current sales job was paying one hundred percent commission. Nonetheless, she went for it and managed somehow.

Skip moved basically across the highway to another upscale neighborhood on the marsh. He could probably, in his golfing days, hit a driver from the Bay Club house to his new rental. It was a much smaller property, but it had a room for each of the kids and all the amenities that Bay Club lacked. However much he tried to adjust, it was not Bay Club. The nights the children were not with him were lonely. He cursed Ashley for making it so. What had our world come to where a father could not live full time with his children? This couldn't be good for society or the nation in the long term—the breaking down of the nuclear family, meaning a mother and father, man and woman, not a Robert and George in a reprehensible relationship. What used to be considered perverted is now the norm in this *Alice in Wonderland* world in which we live.

✝

Skip was lonely and depressed. He took on a teaching job some years ago, thinking that it might be good for him to get back into the world. He taught a few basic business and computing courses at one of the local high schools. He voluntarily took himself off the social security disability. It turned out to be a disaster. His altruistic desire to teach backfired on him in real time. High school was no place for a man with an unstable mind. The administration was unrelenting, the students horrid for the most part, and the day-to-day mental and physical grind on his arm wore him down. Skip never gave up on God, though. He thought God was asking him to go into the public schools to help those in need. This never materialized. It was more than Skip could bear. The schedule was the one upside to the teaching position. He started early, which was not great, but he finished early as well, which allowed him to pick the kids up from school each day—something most parents are unable to do. The days of Mom at home waiting on Johnny to come home from school with milk and cookies seemed to be long gone. It seems that for various reasons, families need that second maternal income to make ends meet, and this takes its toll on the children. Divorce plays its part as well. Skip remembered that if he had a class of twenty-five students, on average, twenty of them came from broken homes. He could see it in their eyes as well as in their behavior. There was listlessness and a sense that no one really cared or nothing really mattered. He wondered what their home lives were like, but he had a good clue. Skip would be able to reach the occasional child with encouragement and a word about God or West Cooper or something nonsecular. He was careful not to stir up too much religious conversation, as it was frowned upon by most and was forbidden by the administration. Even though the law in South Carolina allowed teaching the Bible as a book of history, it was still a slippery slope to actually pull it off. Skip occasionally taught a keyboarding class and would, from time to time, have them type the Lord's Prayer or some other passage from the Bible. He just felt too stifled to come out of the closet with more of an aggressive religious approach. As Mimi used to say, "Bring back prayer in the schools and you will fix everything."

That and a little bit of discipline would go a long way to taking back our school system.

✝

It just kept getting better. It was late August and school was to start the following week. Caroline would be a senior in high school, and Foster would be making his middle school debut. In a conversation with Caroline, she mentioned that Mom is going on vacation in two days to Australia. Skip thought that was peculiar, so he called Ashley to see what was going on. The response on the other end sent Skip reeling once again. Ashley was not only going to Australia with her new boyfriend, unbeknownst to Skip, but her new boyfriend was the man who bought the Bay Club house from them! The audacity of this woman to not only miss the beginning of school and soccer season for Foster and cheerleading for Caroline, but to be in with the new owner of the house she lived in with another man for almost twenty years. Skip's mind started to spin with all sorts of wild notions. Did this guy and Ashley plan the sale of the house? How long had this relationship been going on? After all, Ashley, the good Christian, and Skip had never formalized a separation nor had they been divorced. Another blow to the gut. How many times can one man be brought low? Skip had so many issues that he was in different stages of grief for different mental problems. He hung up the phone and cried in disbelief. Australia. Another man. The house they raised their children in for almost twenty years.

Skip was a man on the ropes. He was at the edge and near the breaking point. He went over to Bay Club to confront the man from Australia with bat in hand. For his sake and Skip's, no one was home. Skip left a scathing note belittling the man and telling him of Ashley's past. That evening Skip was visited by a few of Charleston's finest and told that a restraining order was being placed against him, and he was no longer to go to that particular Bay Club property. The irony. Skip would never again be able to visit the home where he raised his children. He was so bitter against Bay Club that he wouldn't go back there under any circumstances anyway—the final bit that sent Skip to the medicine cabinet looking for something that would stop the pain.

It was fall and Thanksgiving was quickly approaching. Skip wasn't sure what the plans would be with the children. He wondered to himself how many hopeless souls were going through the same situation right now, the possibility of not spending a holiday with one's children. It turned out that Ashley had her mother and husband in for the holiday. Also included in their Thanksgiving at the Bay Club house were Caroline, Foster, and the new man. Skip wanted to take the carving knife to the Australian, and then turn it on himself, but he knew he never could. What was Ashley thinking? That it wouldn't affect the kids having a different man sitting at the head of the table carving the turkey? Skip wasn't sure whether he felt lower during the affair with the other good Christian, or now.

✝

He couldn't return to school for another year. He didn't know it, but it wasn't good for his mental state. He was working on a website for Ashley's lighting business when he stumbled across an opportunity. Skip really hit it off with Peter, the owner of a web design business. It turned out that Peter not only had his own web development business, but he also worked for a large conglomerate and was president of one of the small Internet divisions. One thing led to another, and Peter offered Skip a job and nearly twice what he was making as a teacher. No brainer. Skip gave his two weeks' notice— or was it two days'?—to the high school and was on his way to working on Internet-related projects. But Peter was a different fellow once Skip began to work for him. Skip admired his work ethic and drive and thought that he was an excellent manager. It was just a little more than Skip anticipated. What was once a thriving Internet economy was also caught off guard by the recession that came our country's way. Skip lasted a little less than a year with the company. It seemed appropriate that he was laid off, for he really was in over his head. It was a younger man's game, and Skip had hit fifty and wasn't looking back. There was no animosity between Skip and Peter or the business; it was the way of the world when the business cycle took a downturn. Skip was the first to go, basically due to his large salary catching the eye of corporate management. But he wasn't the last. The division that Peter headed up was slowly dismantled, with most of the small group being let go; a few of the computer programmers landed in some of the other corporate divisions. The whole thing had promise. It got Skip out of the public school system with a big raise. The division was essentially an entrepreneurial arm of the corporation, setting up websites and selling products that ranged from pet beds to baby cribs. The economy got soft and so did their business. So much for happy endings.

✝

Skip had two dear friends, Ann and Bill Brady. Bill was an attorney for a local law firm, and Ann was a mother of three and ran a small court reporting business. They became friends, as often is the case, through their children. Ann and Bill's oldest child was a classmate of Foster's. The boys would get together to watch a football game or go fishing about once a month. Ann knew of Skip's recent layoff and wanted to know if he wanted some part-time work with her court reporting business. Realizing that he had a shortage of income and a lack of opportunities, Skip readily accepted. Skip basically fine-tuned and proofread depositions that Ann had taken. It was pretty straightforward, routine work—just what Skip was seeking.

One afternoon Skip was bringing some documents over to Ann's house so she could take them to an attorney. Ann noticed that Skip didn't look quite right and asked him if everything was okay. For some reason, this was it. This was the breaking point for Skip. Call it a nervous breakdown or whatever you like, but he could no longer control his emotions. Ann brought tissues and a mild sedative for Skip to try to calm him down. He was in such dire straits that she wanted to take him directly to the Medical University to have him checked out. Skip still didn't realize what emotional state he was in, so he decided against going to the hospital. He had visions of Jack Nicholson in *One Flew Over the Cuckoo's Nest* and wasn't ready to go there. Ann pushed hard, as she could see he was in pain. The pain she saw was emotional, not physical this time. Ann made Skip an appointment with a local psychologist and made Skip promise that he would go see her. Skip was reluctant since therapy had never worked for him and Ashley in the past, and he didn't want to go on any type of medicine. He had seen enough medicine in his chemotherapy days. But the appointment was set, so he agreed to go.

✝

Once the dust had settled, Skip purchased a home in an outlying neighborhood in Charleston. This was some feat for a man who had no job or income per se. He used a substantial down payment and the help of Mack and Maria to get into the bank-owned property. It was a lovely one-story house with an additional bedroom over the garage. The house, near the Wando River, had a spectacular river view. Skip liked putting some distance between himself and the Bay Club community, with all its recent notorious memories. The house was perfect for him and the kids. Caroline, of course, assumed the large room over the garage, and Foster took the room closest to the front of the house. Both rooms were painted for them in the color of their choice. Skip had the master bedroom, which left a room for his study and a wonderful sun room that backed toward the river. God had been good to Skip again in allowing the pieces to fall together to make this happen. Another new chapter had begun.

✝

Dr. Lancet seemed all business at first, with a quick welcome aboard and the usual common first-time greeting conversation. Skip saw the couch and wondered if he should lie down on it like in the movies. He decided against it and took an armchair across a small table from where Dr. Lancet sat at her desk. She was a credentialed psychologist with a specialty in post-traumatic stress disorder (PTSD). She came highly recommended by Ann and a few of Ann's friends. It seemed everyone these days had an issue that required therapy.

She asked a few basic questions. Was there any type of addiction or abuse growing up? Skip said no and garnered it was his turn to speak. Skip began at what he thought was the beginning: the cancer. He told her about the fair and getting on the ride with Caroline and breaking his arm. He gave her the *Reader's Digest* version of the radiation and chemotherapy that followed. He said, "If you are wondering why I shook your hand with my left hand, I had limb salvaging surgery that doesn't allow me to lift my right arm." He went through his rehabilitation process, caught his breath, and mentioned the affair that Ashley was having with a coworker at the time. Skip became pretty emotional at this point and began to tear up. No matter how far removed he was as a cancer survivor, the legacy of pain still lived within him. All of this had devastated him to the point of no return. He was letting a lot of this go for the first time really, and it was coming out in tidal waves. The tsunami continued with the more recent events of the separation with Ashley and her escapades with the Australian. He also talked about moving from the Bay Club house and into a rental. Skip mentioned that he had been a teacher but couldn't take it anymore, and so he took the Internet job, only to become unemployed months later. Skip mentioned the possible recurrence of cancer, as *lytic lesions* were found on his latest arm x-ray. Through most of the story, Skip had his head, looking at nothing really, but not looking at Dr. Lancet. He looked up at this point and saw that she had a tissue of her own, dabbing small tears in her eyes. They made eye contact and she said simply, "Your story moves me."

Epilogue

The saga of Skip Sibley ends for the moment. Therapy, family support, a cancer-free body, and hope for the future continue. Skip wanted to find out if there was life after cancer and meet those people and hear those stories that defied the odds. They were not readily available to Skip during his time of need, so he wanted to make sure that those who followed in his footsteps and those who suffered these and similar tragic circumstances knew that there was indeed a light on the other side of the tunnel. While Skip showed many that it's possible to come out of the darkness and step into the light, he wants to emphasize that it's how you react to your new normal that will determine how you go forward.

To finish up with some house-keeping matters, Ashley and Skip were not able to reconcile and divorced in early 2011. The children are older and the relationship between the two is amiable. Skip was able to forgive, but it is the forgetting part that is one factor in his difficulty in obtaining his "new normal." For better or worse, life continues.

Trovo, the family Golden Retriever, made it to around fifteen years old before he went to rest. Like many dogs, it is instinctual to wander to a comfortable place to be for eternity. Trovo found a beautiful spot in the marsh near the Bay Club home where we found him at peace, and buried him at this location. A new black Labrador named Moses is doing his best to fill the shoes of Trovo!

The whereabouts of Ms. Janie still allude the family. It is with hope and desire that Ms. Janie is well and still working her wonderful magic to those in need. Ms. Janie is missed dearly, as she was such a large part of the tough times. Skip hasn't had a sweet potato pie that rivals Ms. Janie's to date.

As far as the current physical health of Skip goes, those lytic lesions were determined to be painful, but not cancerous. This was a great blessing. The mental health side is still at unrest, with peace of mind adverting Skip at most turns. According to his doctors, it may be quite some time before Skip can rid himself, if at all, of the post-traumatic syndromes that caused such pain in his life.

In the end, it is all about faith. Those who have walked down the dark roads know this. Whether they choose to accept God for what he is will go a long way in determining their post-traumatic physical and mental health. Skip wants this story to be one of hope and encouragement, but the tough times must be told openly and honestly. He has walked the same steps as some of you, and in steps not as tough as some of you are going through right now.

The common denominator in all of this is hope in God, for without it, we are all lost souls. As Skip would iterate on his volunteer hospital rounds, "I will pray for your healing on this earth, but your walk on this rock is a short one, so more importantly I pray for your soul to receive grace, and that someday we will see each other in heaven for eternity."

Author's Note

As mentioned in the Prologue, I did my best to reconstruct the pieces of a very true story, my story! In a somewhat humbling way, using the third-person perspective gave me the ability to tell the truth even more so than I could have in the first-person. I fought off the experts and went with a judgment call to write it as so. It is by the grace of God that I had the strength, time, and motivation to finish this book, for which I am eternally grateful. I would particularly like to thank Scott Thomas, who was the original editor of the manuscript. His abilities and omnipresent optimism gave me the courage to continue when times were tough. I would also like to tip my hat to Lisa Kerns, David Phillips, and Jeff Csatari for their editing prowess and encouragement. To the numerous readers, you know who you are; a special thank you goes out to you for also giving me the courage to write this story, and for giving me the hope that someday I could help others by sharing it.

There would be no story without the doctors and hospitals that helped save my life. Roper St. Francis, St. Jude Children's Research, the Medical University of South Carolina, the Washington Hospital Center, and the

Duke Cancer Institute all played significant roles in my healing. To Dr. Angus Baker and his staff for seeing me through to the guiding light, and Dr. Martin Malawer who gave me the ability to continue to have a right arm, thank you. There were many, many more doctors and nurses along the way that provided the ultimate care, too numerous to mention here.

To my children, Langley and Caroline Thomas, and my parents Jack and Rosemary Thomas, I thank you for the love during the dark hours. Please remember that out of darkness comes hope, so keep the faith and don't ever give up the fight.

Made in the USA
Lexington, KY
07 December 2012